A NURSE'S LIFE IN WAR AND PEACE

A NURSE'S LIFE IN WAR AND PEACE

I

This is my usual day for writing letters, and I have nothing but the usual things to write to you about. Each day we get up at the same time, do the same sort of lessons (not very difficult), eat the same sort of food (not very interesting), and go for the same dull walks, with an occasional game of tennis on a badly-kept lawn; but I have been thinking, and the long and short of it is, that I am going to persuade my people to let me leave school.

I think you know that some years ago I determined that I would be a nurse. To be exact, it was in 1883 that Queen Victoria instituted the Royal Red Cross, and in the same year I was grieving over the fact that none of the professions in which my brothers were distinguishing themselves would be open to me, as I was "only a girl"; so I at once decided that I would try to win the Royal Red Cross.

Well, I am not thinking so much about the decoration now, as wars seem to be few and far between; but still I think the nursing profession is the only one I am a bit fitted for, and lately I have been reading everything I can get hold of on the subject.

You see, I am not a bit clever, and I am no good at music or languages; so I could never teach. And, on account of having been so delicate when I was small, I am behind most girls of my age in many subjects; but in the two terms that I have been here I have won two prizes, and I think I can work up any subject that I want to as well as most people can.

I know I am not old enough to begin nursing yet, but when I am, it may be necessary to pay for my first year's training, so I very much want them to save the money they are now paying for my education to pay for that, as it seems to me that I am being stuffed with many subjects that, after I leave school, I shall have no further use for.

I have not yet quite decided which hospital I shall go to. It is clear that if I want to join the Army Nursing Service, I must go in for three years' training in a good-sized General Hospital first; but the best of these hospitals won't accept candidates till they are twenty-three, and that seems such a very long way off. So perhaps I may take a preliminary year in a Children's Hospital, or some other special hospital first, but I am not old enough even for that yet; and as I think F. is going out to the Canary Islands for the spring, I think it is very likely I may go with him, as you know I love travelling.

I like this place very well, and I have many friends here; but one thing is quite definite, and that is that I mean to be a nurse, and with that in view I think I might be employing my time more profitably than I am doing here.

II

PORT OROTAVA, TENERIFE,
April 1889.

Here we are, in comfortable quarters and in glorious sunshine, the grand old Peak of Tenerife (with its cap of snow) looking down upon us.

I wish you could be transplanted to this warmth and brightness; but you would not have enjoyed our experiences on the way here.

You know how cold it was when we left London on the *Ruapehu*; and all down the Channel it was very cold, but fine and calm. We called at Plymouth (such a pretty harbour); then, after we left there, our troubles began. The next day there was a heavy swell, and very few people appeared on deck. Our stewardess, they said, had "happened of an accident," but we were well waited upon by a nice little steward. M. was bad, and stayed in her berth; but with the steward's assistance I struggled up on the upper deck, and I would not have missed it for anything. Towards evening it was really blowing hard, and the waves were grand. We took such plunges down into the trough, and then the great ship trembled, and seemed to pull herself together to rise on the crest of the next wave and then take another plunge.

The men were on the trot all day, making everything fast. It was Sunday, but there was no service—the crew all too hard at work, and the passengers chiefly in their berths. Towards evening I was wondering how I should "make" my cabin, when the purser came along and asked if he might help me down below, as the wind was still rising, and he had been appointed "runner-in" by the captain, who said we had all better be down below.

That night and the next day were really very bad indeed. We were battened down, and the dead-lights were screwed on about 4.30 P.M., and the electric light supply did not come on till after six; so for that time we were in darkness, and some of the passengers were really very much frightened.

Tons of water poured on the main deck and down the companion-ways, and men were bailing it out near our cabins all night long. I kept feeling in the dark to see if there was water in our cabin, as it rushed past the door with a great "swish"; but the step was high, and it did not come over.

There was no sleep for any one that night; it was all we could do to keep from being pitched out of our berths.

The men were very funny as they bailed the water out and mopped up. "Reminds one of washing-day in our backyard—pity my old woman ain't here," "Sometimes we see a ship, sometimes we ship a sea"—and heaps more to the same effect. Our steward said he had never had to bail out so much water before, and he had been six years on the ship. One of the sails was carried away; and when we got to Santa Cruz the engineers discovered that part of the rudder had gone.

Two cooks and one of the sailors were knocked down and injured, but I think not very badly. Two of the boats were washed out of the davits, and one of the heavy deck-seats (next to the one on which I had spent the afternoon) was smashed to bits.

Sleep was quite impossible, as it was most difficult to keep in one's berth, and every now and then there was a great crash as things were broken in the saloons and galleys. We are still bruised and stiff from the knocking about.

I have always wanted to see a storm at sea; but I am now quite satisfied, and I shall never want to see another. It is most unpleasant to be battened down, and the engines sound to be so fearfully on the strain and tremble that you feel you must listen for the next beat of the screw, knowing that if the engines should fail your chance of weathering the storm would be a very small one indeed.

After that the weather improved, and also became warmer, and the passengers one by one came crawling up on deck; but most of them looked as though they had been through a long illness, and could talk about nothing but their alarm in the storm; and the captain owned he had had a very anxious time.

We landed at Santa Cruz early one afternoon—a very unsavoury town, with dirty beggars exhibiting various loathsome diseases and following you about.

After a little delay we secured a carriage and three horses to drive across the island to Orotava, twenty-six miles distant—a pretty, winding road, cool up in the hills, but becoming hot as we descended to Puerto Orotava. The hotel was full, but we secured rooms in a dependence; and when we had rested and changed, we found a *carros* ready to take us across to dinner. A carros is a kind of sledge on broad runners drawn by two oxen. They are much used in the town, as the roads are paved with little cobbles, which would pull the wheels about a great deal.

This is a nice hotel, cool and airy, and the garden is lovely—such quantities of roses, bougainvillias, and bright trees of hibiscus. There is a good billiard-room we can use, and it is open all down one side (only matting blinds). That shows how dry the climate is, as the table is perfectly "true."

The waiters are Spaniards, who know a little English and like to use it. "This is jarm, very goot," &c. We go about with our little red book of phrases, and sometimes get what we want, but more often fail to make ourselves understood. The natives are most interesting, the children such pretty little things with very bright eyes. Up in the hills they still consider it is winter, and the men go about with blankets tied round their necks; and when they squat down on the ground, the blanket flows out and makes a little tent round them. Down here it is really hot, and the small children wear nothing but a little chemise. The women are pretty, and they wear brilliant-coloured handkerchiefs tied over their heads.

We are close to the sea, and it is such a gorgeous blue; I have never seen anything like it before. I suppose it is very deep round here, and the Peak rises 12,000 feet, straight from the sea.

There is no English church yet, but the chaplain holds services in a large room fitted up as a church. Every one rides when he goes anywhere here, even when going to church; so during service there is a large company of ponies and donkeys outside, with the attendant men and boys (all in white suits, with bright-coloured sashes), and now and again the donkeys lift up their voices.

I have found a good chestnut pony ("Leaña") that goes well. They are sure-footed little beasts here; and it is necessary for them to be so, as there is only one "made" road, and for the rest we scramble up mountain paths. But when we get on the road they simply scamper along.

M. has not done much riding; and sometimes, when we are scrambling up a steep place, I look back, and find her holding on for dear life with a most resigned expression on her face. But I think she is enjoying it all immensely.

We walked up to the Botanical Gardens the other day, and they are perfectly beautiful—arum lilies and many of our choicest greenhouse flowers growing like weeds, and the ferns here are so beautiful too. Up in the kloofs (here called *barrancos*) we find maidenhair growing wild, and in such enormous fronds. I measured one, and it was two feet high. At the gardens a very handsome young gardener—a Spaniard—gave us huge bunches of roses to bring away. All the natives we come across are so polite and friendly (every man you pass raises his hat), we wish we could talk Spanish to them; but so far, if we can ask for what we want, it is quite as much as we can manage. The better-class people often speak French, and I get horribly mixed. The other night a solemn señor asked me if I spoke French, and I said, "*Un très mui poco*"!

The word they seem to use the most is *mañana* (to-morrow); as our nice waiter explained when a gentleman said, "Antonio, the coffee is cold," "Ah, it shall be hot to-morrow. With the English it is always now, to-day; with us it is *mañana*."

We hear that Laguna is the fashionable resort as soon as it becomes too hot down here, but that Icod is the fruit-growing village of the island; so we think of driving over and spending a night there.

III

SS. "Fez," English Channel,
June 1889.

Since my last letter we seem to have been chiefly engaged in wrestling with steamship companies in the vain endeavour to persuade them to remove us from the island. F.'s leave was up early in June, and as we had return tickets by one line, we wrote to them in good time to secure berths. At first they made us various promises; but soon we learnt the truth—namely, that all their boats were full in every berth long before they came near the island.

Then we began to tackle other lines; but, you see, nearly all the boats come from New Zealand or the Cape, and this is the favourite time for going home; also there is the attraction of the Paris Exhibition. So I cannot tell you on how many ships we have applied for berths, and always in the end received the news, "Every berth full."

Personally I did not mind, as I enjoyed every day on the island; but it was awkward for some things, and eventually we had to decide to sail on board a small cargo steamer that calls at Orotava instead of at Santa Cruz, and carries a few passengers home at a leisurely speed. But before I tell you of the voyage, I must tell you a little about our last few days on the island.

One day we drove over to Icod, a pretty little village about two hours' drive from Orotava. Much coffee is grown at Icod, and also plenty of fruit— oranges, lemons, figs, &c. We rode from there to Gerachico (a pretty ride along the shore), where a whole village was engulfed when the Peak last erupted; but it is now again built over, and we could not see much of interest remaining.

Señora Carolina reigns at the small Icod hotel, and made us very comfortable. But neither she, nor any one we met in the place, spoke any English; so it was good practice for us, and our Spanish came off better than I thought it would.

We decided not to climb the Peak, as you cannot do it from Orotava without spending a night somewhere up the mountain; but one day M. and I joined a party for a day on the Cañadas—the range from which the Peak rises. We mounted our ponies at 7 A.M. in brilliant sunshine, and at different points picked up our friends, till we were a party of ten, with a crowd of attendant boys to carry our lunch, &c. The first part of the ride was easy and pleasant; then, as we got higher, it became more of a scramble over loose stones, that any English pony would have said were only fit for a goat to be asked to walk over. Just as the path was becoming really steep we left the sunshine, and found ourselves in a thick bank of clouds, cold and damp, and had to go very cautiously, in single file. The chattering pony-boys were very silent (their spirits are easily damped), and said it was "*mucha frio.*" Soon we emerged above the clouds into a scorching sun, and, finding a piece of fairly level ground, some of us took a little canter to try to get warm; but we came to a sandy place, and there Leaña took it into her head to lie down and roll. I saw what she was up to, and managed to roll out of her way; so my saddle was more damaged than I was. But as my clothes were very wet with the mist, the sand adhered!

We had a pleasant lunch, at a height of 8000 feet, while the ponies were off-saddled and fed; and some of us thought we should like to camp for the night and climb the Peak in the morning. But when we had finished lunch we had only two ham-sandwiches left between us, so concluded we had better return before night.

The view was lovely, looking *over* the banks of snowy-white clouds to the very blue sea, with the other islands in the distance, and behind us the grand old Peak.

The ride down (a different way) was rather perilous, the ponies jumping from rock to rock in a perfectly marvellous way, often just on the side of a precipice. But it was too much for some of our party, and they insisted upon walking down; and this rather delayed us, as they could not go nearly so fast, nor were they so sure-footed as the ponies.

We got in at 8 P.M., very tired and very sunburnt, but having enjoyed the day immensely; and our ponies were quite fresh, and wanted to gallop all the way directly they got on the road.

I don't think I have told you about the tree-frogs; they make such a noise after sundown you might think there were thousands of ducks quacking. A gentleman wanted to take some back to England with him; so one day we caught half-a-dozen for him, and they all escaped in our rooms! Such a hunt for them! And I could not finish telling you about Orotava without one word about the *fleas*. They are really a great trial, and seem to abound everywhere, especially in the carriages.

After various false alarms our little steamer, the *Fez* (560 tons), arrived, and began to take in a cargo of pumice-stone. The solemn old oxen brought the carros for our baggage, and our many friends escorted us down to the jetty, where most of the Spanish population seemed to be collected to see us off.

It is always a difficult landing at Orotava, and the small ship's-boat gave us a good tossing before we were hauled up the gangway. It was rather horrid before we got away, and I was the only lady who was not sea-sick before the anchor was up!

Such a change from the *Ruapehu*! Just one very small saloon, and our cabins very tiny; no upper deck, and very little room on the main deck; of course, no doctor on board, and no stewardess. But it was only for a short time, we thought, and we were determined to make the best of things, and soon found there were compensations—namely, a charming captain, nice crew, and most attentive stewards. And very soon my small deck-chair was established on the bridge, and I learnt more about navigation than I should have learnt in years on a liner. There were twelve of us passengers (all people we knew), and twenty-two officers and crew; also a big dog, and a sheep who occasionally strolled into our cabins, until nearly the end of the voyage, when the meat hung up in the stern (there was no refrigerator on board) had run low, and then one day I saw a sheep's skin being washed over the side! There were also many noisy cocks and hens, and a few ducks; and, last but not least, swarms of rats! I had some sugar-cane in my cabin, and the rats rather fancied it; and when I threw things at them to make them go away, they would sit on the cabin doorstep to wash their faces and lick their lips!

We had lovely weather as far as Madeira. When we got there we found it was a public holiday, and we should have to stay three days, as there were

300 pipes of wine to be got on board, and the natives would not work on the holiday. This gave us a good opportunity to see the island, and it was very enjoyable. It is far more green than Tenerife, but I should say the climate, though very mild, is not nearly so dry.

The captain arranged a very nice trip for us to a part of the island that is not often visited by people who call only at Funchal.

We had to get up in the middle of the night, and go on board a small launch (that takes the mails round the island) at 2.30 A.M. It was beautiful moonlight, and Funchal looked very pretty as we steamed away round the great Loo Rock. We reached Caliette at 5 A.M., and had to whistle for some time before the people woke up and brought a small boat out for us.

They made us some coffee, and we had breakfast, and then got into hammocks slung on long poles; and two men carried us up and up the hills till we came to a weird tunnel, which we went through by the light of pine-torches, and emerged in the most grand scenery—rugged hills and beautiful waterfalls, such very vivid greenery everywhere. And amongst all the semi-tropical vegetation we came upon one bed of English forget-me-nots that was most refreshing.

We lunched and rested for some time by a beautiful waterfall, called, I think, "Rabacal"; and then going down it was very hot, and, in spite of the steepness of the paths, some of us slept in the hammocks as we jogged along. The men carried us about twenty-five miles in the course of the day, and did not seem at all tired. But there was a little competition to carry me, as I was the lightest of the party! We got back to Funchal about 9 P.M., and were quite ready for bed.

Owing to this delay at Madeira (on account of the general holiday) the voyage is taking much longer than usual, and by the time we get in—or hope to get in—we shall be fourteen days out from Orotava, instead of the five days we took from London to Santa Cruz. In consequence of this the provisions are running rather low, and a few things have quite run out; but I have enjoyed the voyage immensely.

Before I return home, I hope to visit two or three Children's Hospitals in London, to be interviewed by the matrons, so as to settle where I will go to begin training. I am not old enough for admission to a General Hospital yet.

IV

CHILDREN'S HOSPITAL, LONDON,
June 1891.

I thought I would wait till I had been here three months before writing to tell you of my raw probationer days. At first it was all so very new to me that it seemed very, very hard; and I really think that, if it had not been for the fact that one of my brothers had bet me that I should give it up in a fortnight, I should have done so in the first week. But I rarely bet, and when I do, I like to win! And having had to wait so many years before I could persuade a matron that I was old enough and strong enough, I really could not lightly give it up.

By the end of my month on trial I began to feel my way, and was quite certain that I wished to stay on if they would keep me; and though they were not enthusiastic in telling me my services were invaluable, their only cause of complaint appeared to be that I was slow. So they were graciously pleased to accept my fifty-two guineas (in instalments), and for that sum to allow me the privilege of working hard and fast for an average of eleven hours a day (paying for my own laundry, and buying my own uniform) for the period of one year.

I don't think I was slow in attending to the children; but at first a very large part of one's time is taken up with cleaning and housemaiding—sweeping, dusting, scrubbing, polishing the brass taps and bed-knobs, and washing the children's pinafores and bibs, &c.

When I began, I hardly knew the difference between a broom and a scrubbing-brush. I knew nothing of the labour-saving properties of soda and Hudson's soap, and I don't think I had ever dusted a room; so I did not know how fond the dust was of collecting on the top of screens and pictures and window-ledges, and it took me time to discover these things.

At home our breakfast-hour had always been 9 A.M., and, except for a day's hunting, there were very few things that excited my interest before that hour; so I expected to find it difficult to have had my breakfast and to be ready to go on duty at 7 A.M. But in looking back upon my first week in hospital, the thing that impressed itself upon me more than the trouble of early rising was the fact that during that first month I was always hungry! I have got over the difficulty now, as a weekly parcel of "tuck" arrives from home; and when this comes to an end, I buy some potted-meat or (if funds are low) some plain chocolate to carry on till the next parcel arrives. Nearly all the nurses either have food sent, or else buy a good deal. Of course I did not know this would be necessary, and had not got money at first. And there are a few nurses who cannot afford to buy, but of course we share with them.

Dinner is at 6 P.M., and that is the best meal of the day, as the Matron sometimes comes to it; so the meat is generally well cooked. It is always a scramble to get lunch some time between ten and twelve, and it is not interesting—just chunks of cold meat, and (every other day) bread-and-treacle. Our butter is issued to us twice a week—¼ lb. in a little tin mug—and we have to carry this mug about, for meals in the dining-hall and in the ward kitchen, for as long as it lasts. But if you don't keep a sharp eye on your mug, it often becomes empty in the first day or two, and you stand a good chance of having to eat dry bread for the days before the new butter is put out. I very much dislike coffee; but there is nothing else provided for breakfast but coffee and a loaf of stale bread, and our own butter (if we have any left), so we don't seem to start the day very well. For the rest, we make tea twice a day in the ward kitchens, and can use the ward bread. If funds are high and the lunch bad, we sometimes indulge in rashers of bacon; sometimes on Sunday we have a sausage or two; but it is more usual to fill in the cracks with tea and cake.

Up to now I have been working in a medical ward of twenty-one cots. The sister has charge of a surgical ward as well, and I think she prefers the surgical work; so we don't see very much of her, except when the physicians go round, or when we have very bad cases in. I like her very well, but she is rather stiff; and most of the information I am picking up is from the staff nurse and from the house physician, who is most kind in explaining the reasons for the various symptoms we notice in the cases, and what results he hopes for in the treatment he prescribes.

We had a very sad case in the other day. A working man brought in a little chap of two, called Stanley, very ill with pneumonia and rickets. He said his wife was in another hospital (for an operation), and he had to go to work and leave all his children in charge of the eldest, a boy of ten; and his wife had been so very ill he had had to go to see her in the evenings, and so had not noticed how ill Stanley was. At first he kept holding out his arms to me, and calling in such a piteous little voice, "Lady, lady"; but he soon got quite contented, only every day weaker and weaker. His quiet, patient father came every evening and sat by him, and his mother was to come to see him as soon as ever she was well enough; but the poor woman was too late, and when early one morning she arrived in a cab with a nurse from the hospital, he had just been carried down to the mortuary, and we could only take her to see him lying there, looking very sweet, with some white lilies in his hand.

Then we have dear Philip in. He is tubercular, and *such* a pretty boy; but I think he is too good to live. I am afraid his mother drinks, and he has a rough time of it at home; but his father is a very nice man. Here we all spoil him, as he is really very ill, but is always so patient and bright. He has a mop of brown curls and the smile of an angel. He is one of the few children of the slums who always insists upon kneeling up to say his prayers; and though sometimes he has so little breath to spare that I have to say the words for him, he just kneels there and smiles when I get hold of the words he wants to help him out.

As a contrast, another of my patients was Samuel Abraham, the very ugliest little scrap of skin and bones you ever saw. When he came in he was seven months old, and weighed only eight pounds. He was in for six weeks, and absolutely refused to put on a single ounce. Then every one got tired of Samuel, and as I had not had a turn at feeding him, he was handed over to me; and, more by good luck than by good management, he began to improve, and at the end of my first week he had put on six ounces, and since then he has steadily gained in weight, and begins to look more like a baby than a monkey. He went home the other day, and I wonder much whether his poor mother will be able to rear him, as I am sure he will miss the hourly attention he has had here. We should have kept him longer; but we had three cases of scarlet fever, and they had to be sent to the Fever Hospital, and all the children who could be moved had to go home, and the ward will be sulphured. But I am writing this letter as I sit in the bare ward beside one poor little boy called Jackie, who is so desperately ill with meningitis that they don't like to move him. It is a curious case. Jackie belongs to well-to-do people, and his illness was caused by a fall out of a mail-cart. His head is so retracted that it really nearly touches his buttocks, and he lies in a stiff backward bow. He is quite unconscious, and I have to feed him with a nasal tube; his temperature goes up to 104 and 105.

At first I was rather nervous at being "special" with him, as I have been here only three months, and I have never seen a case like this before; and the sister may not come in to see me, as she has to go into the surgical ward, and we may still be infectious. But of course I can ask her advice about anything, and the house physician comes in twice a day, and is most kind. He assures me no one could possibly do more for Jackie than I am doing. I think he will be moved to a small ward to-morrow (if he lives so long), and then I expect I shall have to disinfect, and very likely go to a surgical ward.

V

I know it is a long time since my last letter to you, but really the days are so full of work there seems to be no peace for letters; and at night one is so weary that, after a wrestle to obtain a bath, one feels fit for nothing but bed. And when I get to bed I feel obliged to take my anatomy and physiology books and do a little study, as the residents are very good about giving us lectures, and I should hate not to do decently in the exams.

I think when I last wrote we had just closed the medical ward (whose Sister had had the honour of beginning my hospital education), and after a few hours off duty I was sent up to a surgical ward on the top floor, next door to the theatre.

I went up rather in fear and trembling, as it was noted for being the hardest ward in the hospital—as the nurses were responsible for the theatre as well —and I didn't see how I could squeeze more work into the days than I had been doing on the medical side. But I received a nice welcome from the sister, and soon found that she was one of the best. She didn't wait for us to do things wrong, and then scold us; but she took pains to show us the *best* way to do them, and then woe betide those who didn't do their best!

I shall always remember my second morning up there, when she said, "Nurse, your bathroom looks very smart and nice." It was the first time a Sister had given me a word of praise, and from that day I didn't mind how hard I worked to please her. There was a different atmosphere about that ward, and I soon felt better in it. The children, too, were a more cheery set. Some of them were very ill; but we did not get the poor little "wasting" babies, and it was very seldom we had a child who minded a noise, so that the boys (at certain hours of the day) could be allowed to sing all the popular songs of the day; and they were a very merry crew. Many people think it must be very depressing to see so many sick children; but, as a matter of fact, the children have very little pain—or, at any rate, only for a very short time—and many of them are enjoying a better time than they have had in their lives before. They are kept clean and warm, and have plenty of good food and plenty of toys to play with, and people who understand them when they have a pain, even when they can't explain where it is.

There have been many changes since I came here. Several nurses who came after I did have already left, and one has gone away ill. I had been in the surgical ward only a fortnight when I was unlucky enough to pick up influenza, and was sent to bed, with another nurse, in a small quarantine-room up above the measles ward. They were rather suspicious as to whether we had scarlet fever, as there was still some in the hospital; so no one was supposed to visit us except the home sister. Her visits were few and far between. Poor thing, she was stout, and the stairs were many! We both felt pretty bad with high temperatures, and should have come off badly for attention if it had not been for the "measles nurse," who had only two convalescent children, and she used to break the rules and come up to look after us. One day she had run up with an offering of buttered toast, when we heard a door open downstairs, and *felt* that the Matron was coming. Nurse vanished into our little kitchen-pantry; but there was no escape from that without passing our wide-open door, and, besides, the Matron was sure to call upon the measles ward on her way downstairs. The buttered toast was stowed away under the bed-clothes, and we were trying to be calm and answer Matron's enquiries as to our health, when we heard a rattling of the hand-lift on which our food was sent up from the kitchen, and we realised that nurse had determined to crawl into that, and so descend to her post of duty. With much alarm we heard the lift go down, and trembled lest the unaccustomed weight should cause it to go down with a run. Matron must have thought us very distrait; but we pleaded severe headaches—a plea that was true enough—and she soon went away, "hoping we should shortly be fit for duty again." We were very thankful when nurse appeared to report her safety, with nothing worse than a crushed cap and a crumpled apron, which had been severely commented upon by the Matron.

They were short of nurses, so as soon as I could get about I went on duty again, and had a nice welcome back to my ward. But it happened to be very heavy just then with several small babies, and two of them had hare-lips that had been operated upon, and it was most important that they should not be allowed to cry at all. So one evening I was sitting in the ward cleaning some instruments that had been used in the theatre for a nasty case of mastoid abscess, and one of these babies began to whimper. I jumped up to subdue it, and in doing so I had the bad luck to prick my thumb. The baby soon settled down again, and then Sister came in and cleaned and dressed my thumb; but in a few days I was in for a badly poisoned hand, and it had to be opened in several places by the house surgeon. He wanted me to be off duty, and out-of-doors as much as possible; so Sister arranged to give me some extra off-duty time, and was awfully kind in doing part of my work for me. But when she told Matron about it, Matron said, "Nurse has been off duty over a week with influenza. If she has to go off again, she had better go home and stop there, as she is not strong enough for the work." But Sister didn't want me to go, and fortunately the ward was getting lighter, and I could keep the babies quiet even with my arm in a sling; so I did what I could, and was sent into the kitchen when the visiting surgeon went round, lest he should order me away. The house surgeon was furious with the Matron about it, but he looked after me well, and though my arm was very painful for a fortnight, and allowed me very little sleep, it soon improved. But my thumb is still stiff and unbendable, and the house surgeon is afraid it will always be so, as he had to cut into it so deeply.

I must tell you about a quaint child we had in about that time. She was a little Irish girl called Kathleen, with a mop of red hair and a pretty little face, but with very crossed eyes. Kathleen was five years old, but had never walked, as her legs were badly deformed; but she got about at a great pace on the floor in a style of her own invention. You never quite knew where you were with Kathleen. She had a very sharp temper; but she was devoted to Sister, and was obedient to me. But any directions given to her as to her behaviour by other nurses were received with scorn and entirely ignored; and if Sister and I happened to be off duty together, on our return we generally had to remonstrate with the child for some piece of naughtiness, and then she would soon be sobbing and penitent.

One day I was off in the afternoon, and when tea-time came Kathleen was missing. They searched everywhere for her; and Matron, who happened to pass, joined in the search. Eventually she was found shut up in the Sisters' dining hall, very much engaged with the food-cupboard. The butter had all gone, so had most of the sugar, some of the biscuits, and, when discovered, she was just drinking up the vinegar with relish. Matron remarked, "A good toffee mixture!" And then she spent half-an-hour trying to make the child say she was sorry, but without success; so she smacked her, and sent her to bed! On my return, of course, I had an account of Kathleen's misdoings, and thought it better to take no notice of her. All the evening as I did my work the little white-faced thing sat up in her cot watching me go up and down the ward, with her poor crooked eyes quite dry; but when the children were all settled for the night and the lights turned down, I went to her, and she flung her arms round my neck and sobbed out, "I *am* sorry, and I won't do it never no more. But I wasn't sorry to that woman, and I don't care if she does smack me; but I shall tell my mother when I go home." Then I lifted her out of her cot to warm her toes by the fire, and after a long talk I extracted a promise that she would tell Matron she was sorry next day; and in a very few minutes she was fast asleep.

I expect that I shall be moved from this ward very soon, and I shall be very sorry. The work is hard and fast, but Sister works as hard as we do; so we are very happy together, and I feel I am getting on.

I have got used to the theatre work too, and (after much labour) have learnt the names of all the instruments in common use, so that I can hand them as they are asked for; and sometimes I am trusted to put out what I think will be required for an operation, and when Sister looks them over she doesn't often find anything missing.

VI

Soon after I last wrote I was sent down to the Out-Patients' Department—quite a different kind of work, and I shouldn't like it for long, but it was interesting for a time.

The numbers vary a great deal. From fifty to a hundred children may be brought up in one day, and many of them require small dressings to be attended to. Then, on two afternoons in the week, the surgeons do small operations; and sometimes there are half-a-dozen children all recovering from anæsthetics at the same time, and all requiring to be carefully watched.

There is a dear old Sister in charge, and one afternoon a week we go out together to visit any special hip cases that are being treated in their own homes, after having been in-patients here. *Such* slums we sometimes have to go to; and yet it is wonderful how nicely the poor mothers keep these children when they are just shown the right way. We have one jolly little chap, who has been for two months in an extension apparatus rigged up on a big perambulator, with the weight hanging over the handle. He has improved so much that they will soon wheel him up in his bed-carriage, and I think the doctor will then sign his release from the extension.

Some of the nurses had rather a joke the other day—a joke which had good results for the rest of us. There is a confectioner's shop near here which we largely patronise, and these girls who were on night duty were hungry as usual, and they went into this shop for tea and scones before going to bed. While they were there, our secretary superintendent came in; and afterwards Mrs. —— (who is quite a friend of ours) told the nurses that, seeing them there, he asked her whether many nurses were customers of hers; and she, pretending not to know him, said, "Oh yes, sir; but we gets more nurses from the Children's Hospital than from any of the other hospitals round here. You see, they feeds them *that* badly there!" I believe he went straight back to the hospital and made inquiries about our food, for not many days after we had bacon for breakfast; and now there is always *something* besides the bread put on the table, and we find it a vast improvement.

Another thing has happened which has helped us considerably. A new nurse has joined, who is a cousin of the senior surgeon. She is an awfully nice girl, but does not look very strong, and after a week or two she retired to bed with a strained back (not very bad). Then her cousin visited her, and then he visited the committee; and it seems they had no idea we had to carry all the big lotion bottles up from the dispensary, and the heavy blocks of ice from the basement, and that we had to drag down the great bags of soiled linen to the basement and then along a lengthy passage—no joke on the doctor's day, when all the twenty cots have clean sheets and counterpanes, &c. So now the porters do these things for us, and we mournfully regret that we were not clever enough to arrange for one of our number to strain her back at the beginning of our training, instead of nearly at the end; but without a senior surgeon for a cousin it might not have paid! Nurse is nearly well again now, and she has asked me to spend part of my next free Sunday with her at the house of this same senior surgeon. I shall be horribly shy, but I can't well refuse.

My brother H. has come to live in town now, and it is very nice for me. He is reading for an exam., and has rooms in Barnard's Inn—such a funny old rookery near Holborn, and not far from here. He stands me a good dinner about once a week, when I am off in the evening; and in return I darn his socks for him, try to take him to church on Sundays, and report his doings in my letters home, so that he need only send them occasional post-cards!

While I was in the Out-Patient Department I was supposed to have my Sundays free, unless an "extra" was especially wanted anywhere; and one Saturday evening I was preparing to go away for the night, when a message came that the night sister was not well, and Matron (who was going away till Monday) wished me to go on duty for her for the two nights. That was about 6 P.M.; so I went to lie down for a bit, and at 10 P.M. the home sister gave me the report and the hospital keys, and I took charge, feeling rather important, but also rather a fraud, as several of the charge nurses then on night duty had been here for many years, and knew far more than I did.

However, we got on very well together, and I rather enjoyed running round to the different wards, and helping with the bad cases.

There was one especially sad case—a girl of ten who had been frightened by rats when left locked up in a house. She had chorea so badly that we had to let her sleep on a mattress on the floor, and it was most difficult to keep any clothes on her, or to feed her. Poor child, her temperature gradually rose till it reached 107.8 before she died, a few days later. The doctors said it was the worst case they had ever seen, and I hope I may never see another case die of chorea.

On the Monday morning I went to bed at 5 A.M., and had to be on duty in the Out-Patient Department at 8 A.M. We had a heavy day; and when we finished at 5.30 P.M., you can imagine my disgust at receiving a message from Matron that I was to relieve the nurse who was in quarantine with a whooping-cough case, from 6 to 10 P.M. I was very glad the child whooped fairly often, as otherwise I should probably have gone to sleep.

The next morning I *did* over-sleep, and was ten minutes late for breakfast, thereby incurring a lecture from the Matron; but I could not refrain from remarking to her that I had had only two hours' sleep since Sunday (until that night), and she said, "What *do* you mean, Nurse?" And then it came out that when she sent me to quarantine she had quite forgotten that I had been on night-duty for those two nights, but I had to relieve in quarantine again that night in spite of it. Of course none of us ever mind doing extra duty when it is necessary, but there were plenty of others who might have done it, and got their full amount of off-duty time as well.

Since then I have been working in several different wards, and there are so many new nurses who have come since I did, that I am generally first probationer now, and it is far more interesting, and when the staff nurse is off duty, I take her place.

Matron has been quite civil to me lately, so I suppose my reports have been all right, as I believe she disliked me very much at first, and did not take much trouble not to show it.

Just now I am again in the Out-Patient Department, as Sister has been called home on account of illness, and I am working it with another probationer, and with no sister. The other probationer is two weeks senior to me, but she has not been down in the out-patients before, so we are not quite clear which of us is in command; at present I make her take the lead on medical days, and I do on the surgical days, as I am more used to the surgeons and their ways; and we get along very well.

I shall very soon have finished my year here, and have been very much exercised over the question of what I had better do next.

One of the sisters that I have liked here has been appointed Matron of a small Children's Hospital, and she has offered me a post as Staff Nurse. This was very kind of her; but, on the whole, I think I would rather get my adult training before I do anything else, as I am afraid it would be rather hard to begin at the beginning again, if I went on to being a staff nurse with children.

The Matron advises me to take a good long rest before beginning in an adult hospital, as I have got very thin and run down of late, and I am still a year too young to be received at the best hospitals; so it is just possible I may accept an invitation from my eldest brother to go out to him for a year in South Africa.

In the meantime, I am gathering all information about the London hospitals, and am to visit two or three of them for interviews with the Matrons before I leave here.

I have passed my exams. all right, so my first certificate is fairly safe. For many reasons I shall be very sorry to leave here, but oh! I am so tired, and to think of being able to stay in bed till I feel I want to get up, is a joy indeed.

VII

When I last wrote to you I was still a humble pro., often a weary, hungry, and foot-sore pro., but withal a happy one, and I hope one day to be a pro. again—but for the present, times have changed.

I have come out to stay with my brother, who is the Judge-President here. He has lived here for the last eleven or twelve years, but this year there is a great Exhibition in Kimberley, so he has taken a larger house for the time being, and will be able to entertain a few friends who will be coming up for the Exhibition.

I left Southampton in June, on the R.M.S. *Scot*, and had a very pleasant voyage out in good weather. I suppose people are always especially kind to a "lone lady" on board ship; at any rate, I had a very good time.

There were not many passengers on board, only forty-two gentlemen in the first class, and seventeen ladies, so I had a nice big cabin to myself.

The *Scot* is the only twin-screw steamer on that line, and it was lucky she had a twin screw, as, when I woke up the first morning out from Southampton, there was a strange silence on board, and when I got on deck I found there had been an explosion in the engine-room, and the top of the high-pressure valve was blown off; there was some talk of having to signal for a steamer to tow us into Brest, but after awhile, the engineers concluded they could patch up matters, and we could proceed with one screw working; this reduced our speed, but I did not mind that at all.

The Bay behaved very nicely, and I did not miss a meal in the saloon all the way out. We had a few hours ashore at Madeira while they were coaling and overhauling the damaged machinery, and the flowers and fruit were beautiful as ever; the men and boys swarmed round the steamer in little boats, and would dive into the sea for silver coins thrown overboard: one or two of them could dive down under our ship and come up on the other side.

The next day we passed the Canary Islands, and had a good view of my old friend, the Peak of Tenerife.

We had the usual board-ship entertainments; two dances (the stewards make a very good band), several concerts, an amusing "Trial by Jury" of one of the passengers, sports for the passengers and for the crew, plenty of cricket and other games. This is the programme for one day from my diary:—

Seven A.M.: Salt tub. 7.30: On deck, tramp and talk, and then read. 8.30: Breakfast; excitement over the sweepstakes on the ship's run, &c.; read, prepare programmes for the concert at night, hunt up people to sing, &c.; watch a whale and flying-fish. 12.30: Fire and boat drill by the crew. 1 P.M.: lunch, sleep. 3: play cricket. 4: tea, choir practice, tramp and talk. 6.30: dinner. 8.30: concert, tramp and talk and watch the phosphorescence, and look for the Southern Cross till 11 P.M.; then bed, and as sound a sleep as though I had done a day's work. A sea-voyage, with pleasant people on board, and not too rough a sea, is the most restful way of taking a holiday I can imagine.

It was very damp and hot crossing the Line, and the cabins became so stuffy that sleep at night was somewhat difficult; but one could make up for that by sleeping a few hours in the day when up on deck.

All too soon we anchored in Table Bay, under the shelter of Table Mountain. Many people are disappointed in their first view of Table Mountain, but it has a grandeur all its own, and it grows upon you.

My brother was unable to meet me as he had intended, but a friend of his came on board—a gentleman who was down in Cape Town for the session of Parliament—and I found it was arranged for me to spend a day or two with him and his family at Sea Point, a suburb of Cape Town, before continuing my journey "up country."

Having come nearly 7000 miles alone, it did not seem to make a great deal of odds having to do another 700 miles alone; but I was glad of a few days' rest, with pleasant people.

I had made so many friends on board the ship that it was quite sad to say good-bye to them all; and I had more than one kind invitation to stay with people in different parts of South Africa.

The day after we landed, I was taken to hear a debate in the House of Parliament on the Deceased Wife's Sister's Bill. The people I was staying with went on to a reception at Government House, and wanted to take me with them; but I begged off, not having unpacked suitable garments.

It is very pretty all round Cape Town, and I hope to see more of it before I return home.

Then, one evening at 9 P.M., I was seen off from Cape Town Station, and was once more a traveller on my own account, but not under such comfortable conditions as on board ship. I learnt that the dining and sleeping cars were attached to the trains only on one night of the week (the night the mail-boats come in), so I went in an ordinary first-class carriage, the ticket costing me more than £8, and found the seats were covered with horse-hair, and by no means comfortable for a night journey. Above the seat there is a shelf which lets down at night, so that four people can secure lying-down room in each carriage.

I soon learnt, also, that in this upside-down country, in spite of the fact that it was the month of July, it was also the middle of winter, and as we got up to higher altitudes it became intensely cold. I had the carriage to myself at first, and, having piled on all the clothes I had with me, I was trying to sleep, when, about 2 A.M., two old Dutch ladies were put in with me, and for the rest of the night they chattered, and ate cheese and apples and onions, so that sleep was impossible until they left the train at Matjesfontein.

I am told the scenery we passed through that night is very grand. I hope some time to see it under more favourable conditions.

Cold and hungry, about 7 A.M., we stopped for breakfast at Matjesfontein. I took my sponge-bag and towel, thinking I should find a waiting-room; but all I found was a tap on the platform, where we took our turn at a splash in icy-cold water, and then went on to a tin shanty, where breakfast was served —kippers, good bread, indifferent butter, and moderate tea.

There did not seem to be any hurry; but when we had all finished, and the engine had had a drink, and the engine-driver had lit his pipe, we started off again. And all that day we strolled across the Karroo, stopping (apparently) just when the driver felt inclined, and, when there was a hill, going so slowly one felt tempted to jump off and take a little exercise by running alongside.

It was very grey and brown, this wonderful Karroo country, with occasional kopjes (hills with great boulders of stones up the sides), and now and then a river or a stream, and always by any water a green line of the mimosa trees covered with their yellow flower.

As the sun grew stronger I began to forget the discomforts of the night, and some pleasant Dutch people came on board and told me many interesting things about the country we were passing through. Then I was introduced to my first swarm of locusts; a weird sight it was, too. They were pointed out to me first when they were some miles ahead of us, and looked like a small black cloud; then, as they came near, the sky seemed to become black with them, and we had to shut all the windows or the carriage would soon have been full of them. They tell me sometimes the young ones settle on the lines in such masses, and the lines become so slippery, the trains can't get on, and the men have to turn out and shovel them off. Fancy a Great Northern express being held up by a swarm of locusts!

For most of the way the old waggon-road ran alongside the railway, and was marked out by the skeletons of horses and oxen, or the sadder sight of a mound of stones with a little wooden cross, where some poor fellow had "fallen by the way."

We stopped at Victoria West for dinner; and as there was another train (from up country) in the station, we were halted well out on the veldt, and I had to stumble along to the station, and then, across what seemed in the darkness to be a rickyard, to the tin shanty where dinner was served. I was the only lady there; but I had only had a snack lunch on board the train, and we were more than an hour later than we had expected to dine, so I was too hungry to mind much, and had a very good dinner. There is only a single line for all this long track, so the delays to allow trains to pass at the stations are numerous, and it is well never to travel without a supply of chocolate, as the meals are very movable feasts.

I managed to sleep through that night, as it was not so cold, and I had the carriage to myself. Early the next morning we steamed into Kimberley, and my brother met me at the station.

VIII

Two things are prominent in my mind to-day: the first is that the thermometer is at 104° in the shade, and the mosquitoes are perfectly vicious; and the second is that the Kimberley Exhibition, with its round of gaieties, is actually closed. But before I tell you about this Exhibition, I must try to go back and give you a few "first impressions" of the Diamond Fields.

As you come into Kimberley by train, you first pass the Kaffir Location; and, instead of the picturesque dwellings that one sees in pictures, you see an exceedingly untidy collection of huts built of all sorts of odds and ends —bits of galvanized iron, old paraffin tins, &c. Then come small tin shanties inhabited by the "poor whites"; and so the houses improve, as one nears the centre of the town.

We drove down from the station in a Cape cart, which takes the place of a fly here. It is a comfortable kind of dog-cart with two wheels, drawn by a pair of horses; it has a movable hood, and the four passengers all sit facing the horse's tail. The most comfortable seats are at the back, and part of the driver's seat lifts up on a hinge while you get to the back seat.

I found my brother had taken a house and bought all the furniture in it, so there was not much difficulty about settling in, except hanging our own pictures and buying a little more linen, plate, &c.

It was a nice brick-walled bungalow, with the usual galvanized-iron roof, and a shady balcony (called here a stoep) all the way round the house, so that one could generally find a fairly cool place to sit.

He had also secured a very good white woman as cook, and a dusky Zulu called George, who waited at table, and generally fagged for the cook. George looked about fifteen, so I treated him as I would a boy of eleven or twelve, and he was soon my most devoted slave. But one day I asked him how old he was, and he said, "I was thirty-four last census, missus." But I shall continue to treat him in the same way, as it seems to answer well; and, after all, I think these blacks will always be rather like children, however old they are. I find he has a wife at a kraal, up country, and he is now saving up to buy some cows wherewith to secure another wife. I understand the present value of "a nice Kaffir girl" is seven cows!

There is a large compound at the back of the house; and thrown in with the house we found two dogs, a dignified cat, and some fowls and turkeys.

At first I thought the Kimberley people were rather uninteresting, and felt inclined to agree with the barber who, when he was giving me a most refreshing and much-needed shampoo after the dusty journey up, said, "You *will* think the ladies here funny, miss, for they absolutely never talk about anything but their dresses"; but, poor things, there was very little else to talk about.

Every one was kind in coming to call, and I soon found some very nice people amongst them. Sunday is the great day for all the gentlemen to call; and sometimes we had eight or nine men dropping in on Sunday afternoon, and generally one or two came in to supper after church.

There is a splendid library nearly opposite the club (which is also a fine building), and I very much appreciate the cool reading-room, with all the English papers and magazines, only about a month old.

We play a good deal of tennis on gravel courts. There are two days in the week when ladies can play at the club, and some people who have private courts have regular "days," so that I generally play three or four afternoons a week. Just lately I have had some good riding, as a young lady I know has gone down to the Cape, and has left a nice and young horse behind. Her mother offered to lend it to me one day, and I had a glorious gallop over the veldt with their groom; and then a kind note came, saying that "I was doing them a great favour by exercising the horse, as it was too fresh for the younger girls." I am glad to be able to do a favour so easily, and we make up very pleasant little riding parties.

I think the thing one misses most in Kimberley is water. If you ride or drive, you may find some out at the waterworks or (a variable amount) in the river out at Alexanderfontein, but the water you can find within walking distance might be measured in bucketsful; and the men are fond of talking of the "early days," when it was cheaper to have a bath in soda-water than in plain water, and of a notice that was said to have been put up in a hotel, "Please do not use soap, as the water is required for tea."

In the season, with careful watering, one can grow a good many flowers. Roses do especially well, and some people who are diligent with the watering-pot cultivate a small piece of grass; but a few days' neglect, or a few hours' visitation from a flight of locusts, and your treasured piece of grass is as though a prairie fire had been over it.

Of course there was much excitement up here about the opening of the Exhibition. The Governor and family came up from Cape Town for the ceremony, and stayed nearly a fortnight in Mr. C.'s house—which he gave up to them—and there was much entertaining.

We had the Colonial Secretary and his wife staying with us, and also a daughter of the Governor of Bechuanaland. As Mr. —— was the Minister in attendance on the Governor, he had to bring his secretary with him, and the police superintendent posted a mounted orderly at our gate to take his messages about; so we felt quite important.

Many interesting people from all over South Africa came up for the Exhibition, and I am afraid I shan't be able to remember all those to whom I have been introduced.

Mr. Cecil Rhodes was here for a few days, and we went to supper with him one Sunday evening. He is generally supposed to dislike ladies; but if that is true, he does not show it. There were not many there, and I sat next to him at supper. I believe it was a very good supper; but the conversation was so interesting (all about South Africa and South Africans) I couldn't attend to it, and I went home hungry, and had to have a private snack before I went to bed.

The morning after the Governor arrived we received an invitation to dine at Government House that evening; and it was rather awkward, as we had a dinner party here. But P. and Mr. —— went off to call and explain matters, and we were excused. They gave two huge garden parties, which we attended, and I enjoyed them very much—both the Governor and lady so very pleasant and friendly. Another day they were the guests of De Beers, and we also were invited; so we saw all the process of diamond-mining under very comfortable circumstances: the blue stone as it was brought up from the mines in little trucks and laid out in the sun (surrounded by barbed-wire fences) to pulverize, then collected and crushed and washed; and then we went into the sorting-shed, and were given trowels to sort with, and I found four nice diamonds in ten minutes, and should like to have kept them! then to the packing-room, and saw *such* diamonds, bags and bags of them. Afterwards we drove out to Kenilworth, the model village, all planned by Mr. Cecil Rhodes for the De Beers' men. Such nice little houses, with water laid on, and every convenience; a good garden to each house; a school and a club-house; a recreation ground; and then miles of fruit-trees —grapes, peaches, apricots, &c.—that Mr. Rhodes has planted and has had carefully irrigated. One could hardly believe it was so near to Kimberley, and Kimberley dust.

Every day at the Exhibition there was a good band playing, and every evening some fireworks and other entertainments. Cricket matches—played on a pitch of cocoanut matting—tennis tournaments, &c., were the order of the day; so that now, when the Governor and other visitors have returned to the Cape, and the Exhibition is closed, you can understand that Kimberley seems a little flat, and I am much looking forward to a run down to the Cape next month by way of a change.

IX

KENILWORTH, NR. CAPE TOWN,
January 1893.

Here we are, amidst lovely greenery and flowers, with the turtle-doves cooing in the garden, and with the very blue sea on one side and grand old Table Mountain towering above us on the other.

Kimberley was really a very warm place before we left it. We had had several bad dust-storms, when you shut up all the doors and windows, and still the dust comes through, and settles in inches on the furniture, and everything you touch or taste is dusty.

One of the worst dust-storms, and the hottest of days, was Christmas Day. We had invited a few lonely men to dinner; and when I came in to dress, George met me at the door, and said, "Missus, kitchen window all gone; dinner no good." And when I went to investigate, I found poor Stanley nearly weeping, as the window had been blown completely in, frame and all, on to the table at which she was preparing our dinner; and the dignified cat was licking up the custard on the floor!

Fortunately the turkey was saved, and, with the help of a few extra tins, we scraped together a fairly good dinner. I don't know what would become of the people in Kimberley if they were afraid to eat tinned foods.

Besides the dust (and my old enemies, the mosquitoes), the flies were very horrible. They settle everywhere, and it is necessary to keep everything very well covered up. You have to shoo them off the sugar before you help yourself; and if you venture to put some honey or jam on your bread, it is ten to one there is at least one fly on it before it reaches your mouth!

Well, we left Kimberley still gasping for rain, and the train strolled down to the Cape in two days and one night.

The scenery we passed through on the second day was very fine indeed, all through the Hex River Pass. I saw a good many baboons. One little chap scuttled away, and then sat down and threw stones at us. A most quaint little beast he looked, in a fury of a temper.

Mr. —— met us at the station, and they have such a delightful house and garden. You have no idea what a rest it is to see plenty of greenery again, after all the sun and glare of Kimberley.

All the people about here seem to be so very pleasant and friendly, I am enjoying myself immensely.

We went to dinner one night at Government House. I was shy at the prospect of going, but it was really very jolly. I went in to dinner with Captain —— of H.M.S. —— (now at Simonstown), and he was very entertaining. The men were all in naval, military, or court dress, and they looked so nice.

Another day Mrs. —— gave a picnic at Constantia, the Government wine farm, and the Governor and party joined us there.

It was a very pretty place, and after tea we went for a scramble up a ravine to pick blackberries. Part of the way up I was trying to disentangle Lady —— from a bramble, when the Governor turned round and called to her, "Hurry up, my dear, hurry up!" and she replied, "But, H. dear, I'm caught by my hair." So he had to return to assist; and then coming down he twice fell down, and each time pretended he had sat down only to admire the view!

On Sunday we went over to Simonstown to call on the Admiral's wife. There were two captains of men-of-war calling, and some other officers, and they invited us to visit them on their ships; but P. could not spare a day. I was rather disappointed.

Mr. Cecil Rhodes was away, but we walked over to see his place, Groot Schuur. It is a very lovely and peaceful spot, just at the foot of Table Mountain, and with lovely views in all directions. The hydrangeas that he is so fond of are quite a sight; they grow up the sides of a hollow glen in the grounds, and the mass of different shades is very beautiful.

Another day we went to lunch with the Chief Justice at Wynberg. Such a lovely place he has, with many beautiful trees in the grounds. Amongst others they have a good many of the silver trees which grow up Table Mountain, and, I believe, nowhere else in the world.

In the afternoon Lady —— drove us to a huge garden party at Newlands (Government House). I heard that 1600 invitations had been sent out, and I should think most of them had been accepted. But there was still plenty of room, and the grounds are beautiful; and there was a good band playing. One of Khama's sons was there, but I did not meet him.

My brother was anxious to have a little sea-bathing, so we stayed for a few days at a small place called Muizenberg, on the shore of False Bay. I have never bathed in such deliciously warm water before. I believe there are some sharks around Table Bay, but False Bay is considered quite safe; so many Cape Town people go out there to bathe, and some of them have bungalows near the sea.

I was very keen to climb Table Mountain, so I left P. for one night at Muizenberg, and went to spend the night again at Kenilworth, with some friends who were making up a "mountain party."

We were up early, and left in Cape carts—a party of eight—at 5 A.M., and drove round to Hout's Bay Neck. Most unfortunately it was a cloudy morning, and the mountain is said to be dangerous in a fog; but we kept hoping it would clear, and we began the climb at 6.45 A.M.

It was fairly steep, but never really a difficult climb. When we got to the ranger's cottage, we found he had just killed a horrid cobra snake that measured 5 feet 6 inches long. He did not hold out any hope of the weather clearing; but as we had gone so far, we thought we might as well go on. So we clambered to the top, where we arrived at 11 A.M., and were greatly disappointed not to get any view. The only compensations were the flowers we found, which were simply lovely—huge white heather, and many-coloured everlastings, and many flowers which I had never seen before.

Coming down in the afternoon, it was blowing and cold, and at one place we missed the path, and for about a mile had to force our way through some thick and very wet undergrowth, and then it began to rain. So we were rather a draggled-looking party when we reached the carts, and the drive home in our wet garments was not exactly comfortable.

This may not sound as though we had a very enjoyable expedition, and yet I really did enjoy the day very much. The people were all so jolly, and made fun of all the discomforts.

Major ——, the Governor's secretary, was one of the party, and he had provided himself with pins, needles, bandages, sticking plaster, and all sorts of other things, most of which came in useful in the course of the day. I heard afterwards that he told the Governor that he had never done such a hard day's work before, as we made him walk for eleven and a half hours, and only let him sit down for half an hour!

The time has gone so quickly down here, as there has been so much going on, and every one has been so kind. We have had about twice as many invitations as we could accept.

Now we are packing up to return to Kimberley, and as they have had some good rains up there, I hope we shall find it a little cooled down. If only we could take some of this lovely greenery with us! You have no idea how grateful you ought to be in England that you can always find a green field if you go to look for it, instead of perpetual greyness and brownness and glare.

Soon after we get back P. will have to start off on circuit in the colony, and I am hoping to go part of the way with him, and then to start off on an expedition to visit some friends up country in Natal; they are fifty miles from a railway. I am looking forward to this tremendously. And then soon after it will be time for me to make tracks for home, as I have now nearly reached the venerable age of twenty-three, and am therefore eligible for beginning my training in an adult hospital. And though this sort of life is very jolly for a time, I should not like it for always; it is not so satisfying as useful work.

I am quite sad at saying good-bye to all my friends. I believe one makes real friends more easily out here than one does in England. It must be something in the air.

X

After my last letter to you we journeyed back, over the seven hundred odd miles to Kimberley, and found life up there a little flat after the gay time we had been having at the Cape; but I had some good tennis and riding, and then we had to prepare for the circuit.

At each place that the judge visits he has to do a little entertaining, so he has to take a cook and a butler with him; and as some of the places where courts are held are quite villages, he has to take a certain amount of groceries along too—and, of course, wine.

The Government provide a saloon carriage with a small kitchen on board, so that is used as the judge's headquarters when near the railway lines; but many of the places visited entail long drives in Cape carts.

The first place we went to was Colesberg, and we arrived there at 6 A.M. We were quite a large party with the barristers, the clerk and registrar, the interpreter, and the servants.

We were met by the magistrate and the sheriff, with a smart escort of Cape Mounted Police, and a party of convicts to take the baggage up.

We found a nice little house ready for us, the owner having turned out to make room; and, after a wash and breakfast, the men all went off to the court, and I stayed to unpack and get things straight.

There were three coloured girls left to do the housework, &c. None of them could speak English, and they had several babies scattered about. I knew we had to give a dinner party before we left, and felt rather hopeless about how it would go with the material to hand. However, everything went off very well in the end. Lots of people called on me, and I had some good tennis at the club, and also some nice rides on a horse that was lent to me, the first one I have tried since I came to this country that had a good mouth; most of them are ruined with the bits they use.

The surrounding country was rather pretty, and good for corn and cattle.

We stayed four days at Colesberg, and then moved on to Craddock, ten hours on the railway. There was a lot of court work there, and it had to be fitted into five days; so the men were in court nearly all the time—one night up to 11 P.M.—and I found it a little slow. But I had some nice drives, one day going out to see some curious sulphur baths, and another day to a farm about eight miles off, where every imaginable kind of fruit seemed to grow.

After this we parted company, my brother going on to Middleburg, and I for another run of ten hours in the train to Port Elizabeth, where I joined the *Drummond Castle* for Durban.

Various people seemed to have asked the captain to take care of me, so I sat next to him at table, and he was most kind. When he found that I meant to put up at a hotel in Durban, he told me that he wouldn't let me do that, as he had lots of friends there, and I should have a much better time if I went to stay with them.

We got to East London next day. The sea was rather rough, and there was a lot of cargo to get on board, so we were there some time; but I didn't go ashore. When we had again got under way, the captain came up to me and said, "I have wired to some people in Durban to ask them to meet you when we get there." Was it not kind of him?

When we reached Durban I waited till the captain was ready to go ashore; and then we got into a kind of huge clothes-basket, and were swung over the side and into the tender, as these big steamers can't get into the harbour. And when we had come alongside the wharf, we found two ladies waiting for us, with a sweet pair of cream-coloured ponies.

They assured me it was quite all right, and that they really had lots of room, and the captain was to come up to lunch. So off we drove to such a nice house up on the Berea, with a lovely view right over the harbour.

They were very pleasant Scotch people, and they *were* so kind to me, driving me about to see the town, &c.

I stayed the night with them, and all the next day, as there was no train till 6 P.M.; and then they saw me off, and made me promise to visit them on my way back.

I got to Pietermaritzburg at 10.30 P.M. (I believe it is very fine scenery on the way up, but it was too dark to see it), and stayed a night at a hotel, where I found that my kind Durban friends had wired to the proprietress to look after me; so everything was very comfortable.

I was up early the next morning to have a look round Maritzburg, and made friends with the driver of the post-cart, who promised me the box-seat. "John" was quite a character, and he entertained me well for all the forty-five miles we drove that day.

We got away at 10.30 A.M. with six tough little horses and the funniest old Noah's Ark of a coach you ever saw. The road was very rough, and there were very steep bits down to rivers (or "spruits," as they are called here), and then a hard pull up the other side. We changed horses several times, and some of the teams were very raw and wild; and the leaders were sometimes inclined to turn round and come to see how the shaft-horses were getting on. So John had to use his huge whip at times, and I had to cling on, and I got so bumped about that I was stiff for days afterwards.

John had many interesting stories to tell, having been a despatch-rider for us in the Zulu War.

My friends met me a mile or two outside Greytown with a mule-cart, in which we drove up to their farm—such a delightful old house. It really belongs to Mrs. ——'s father, but he is in England now, where they have some children at school; so they have come up from their smaller house in Greytown to take care of the farm.

I have been here a fortnight now, and have enjoyed every minute of it. For one thing, the climate is delightful. It is pretty hot, but not the damp heat you find near the coast, nor the dusty heat of Kimberley. So I am feeling very fit, and the people *are* so nice I should like to stay for months. It is a very free-and-easy life, and we are waited upon by a man in a shirt and an apron of cats' tails!

It is very pretty country, and I am having delightful rides on a good horse. One day we rode out to see some people who live fifteen miles away from here, and they insisted upon our staying the night. Of course they don't get many visitors out there. The next morning we rode on to a place where we got a splendid view over what they call the Thorne country, right into Zululand. We could see the Mooi River valley, and they pointed out to me where the "defence of Rorke's Drift" saved Natal.

I had never been inside a Kaffir hut, so we went one day to explore; and I was taken to call upon "Sixpence," a Zulu who works here. We had to crawl into the wattle and straw hut on our hands and knees, and at first I could not see anything and could hardly breathe, as the only escape for the smoke from their fire is through the doorway; but we squatted down on the floor—which looked clean and polished with much sitting upon—and soon I made out Mrs. Sixpence (Sixpence can only afford one wife), with a blanket draped around her, and four children. The baby was absolutely naked, and the other children were chiefly clad in beads. And then there was Sixpence's mother, a poor old thing who is over a hundred, and can remember Chaka, the great Zulu chief.

I have collected many curios while staying here, and the other day I was given the skin of a huge python 18 feet long, which had been shot near to the house not long before. I can't bear snakes and creeping beasts, and there are a great many of them up here. There is more grass than there is in Cape Colony, and so better cover for the beasts. The other day, when I was out riding, my horse gave a great jump aside, and after I had remonstrated with him I looked back, and saw a horrid snake sitting up and hissing at us; so I had to explain to my gee how sorry I was that I had spoken!

The doctor with whom I am staying has to take very long journeys on horseback to see his patients. He seems very popular, and often has to go to Kaffir kraals a long way off, though many of the natives still stick to their faith in the witch-doctors and their weird remedies. Very often they have no money, so he is paid in kind; and sometimes he returns from a visit to a chief with one or two cows, which he has to drive home before him.

Several people have asked me to stay with them; and if I was not in such a hurry to get back to work, I am sure I could put in several months up here with much enjoyment, the Natal people are quite delightful, and so hospitable. But John has promised me the box-seat on his Noah's ark again on Tuesday, and I must once more make tracks for Kimberley.

XI

I managed my journey back from Natal very comfortably, and made several new friends on the way.

The drive on the post-cart from Greytown to Maritzburg was somewhat perilous, as there had been a great deal of horse-sickness about, so that good horses were scarce; and several of our teams were very raw, and there was much bucking and kicking before each start; and several times the harness broke down, and John had to descend to make repairs. I am sure the passengers in the body of the ark were terrified lest the horses should take it into their heads to start off while the reins were entrusted to me; and though I am pretty good at managing a horse, I should be shy of trying to drive six of these bucking creatures. However, we got safely down to Maritzburg in the course of the day, and again I had to spend a night there, taking the train the next morning for Durban.

The railway between these two towns is a wonderful piece of engineering work, crawling up one side of a mountain and scuttling down the other; very fine scenery, with sub-tropical vegetation, all the way down.

My good Durban friends again met me, and were most kind, putting me up for the night, and then seeing me off on the *Courland Castle*, rather a tub of a coasting vessel, that gave us such a pitching about that even I succumbed and was sea-sick. This greatly annoyed me, as I had come all the way out to the Cape without a qualm!

I had meant to do a jaunt up from East London to visit some people at Grahamstown and at King William's Town, but I was so happy at Greytown that I stayed on longer than I intended, and had to give up the other visits.

We anchored off East London for some hours, and the captain took me ashore to lunch with some friends of his; and they took us for a nice drive round the town and out to a place called Cambridge, where we picked oranges and lots of flowers. The scenery at the mouth of the Buffalo River is very pretty.

Then we went on to Port Elizabeth, and the captain again took me out to lunch; and we had a pleasant day exploring the town with some of his friends, and in the evening they saw me off by train for Kimberley. The train was rather full, but I was so tired that I slept all night, and woke up only just in time to get some breakfast at Craddock. I am getting quite experienced in making good use of the twenty minutes they allow you to get meals at these wayside stopping-places.

All that day we were strolling along in the train—dinner at De Aar Junction in the evening—and at 4 A.M. the next morning I reached Kimberley. No one to meet me, and no cabs; so I left my baggage with a porter, and walked down to our house. Peter, the cat, was holding an "at home" in the garden, and Carlo, the retriever, was on the stoep to welcome me, and assisted me to find the key under the doormat; and I was glad to find my bed ready to tumble into, after a much-needed wash.

It is winter here now, and the people seem rather more energetic than usual. I have been to two dances since I got back, and there are some dinner parties in prospect.

The other day I went down a diamond mine—a thing visitors don't often do, though, of course, a good many see all the workings above ground. I had to dress up in a canvas overall suit and sou'wester, and then, in a very rough cage, we were lowered to the 1800-feet level. I hear they will soon be working at 2000 feet below the surface, but 1800 feet is the depth they are working just now.

It was all very interesting—swarms of natives (with very little on!), and the fussy little trucks rushing about with their loads of the blue-stone, in which the diamonds are found—but I was rather glad to get back to the daylight again.

Then on Sunday afternoon I was invited to go and see a war-dance by the Zulus in the mine compound. It was really very fine. Only one tribe is allowed to dance at a time, or there would soon be fighting; and the men of the other tribes kept away at the far end of the compound, and would not look on. There were about forty Zulus dancing. They were dressed in little aprons of cats' tails and a few beads, and wore feathers on their heads, and were waving skin shields and knobkerries (sticks with weighted knobs). They all stood in a row, and stamped, and clapped, and danced, and sang in very good time; and then single ones stalked out in front of the others, and, throwing themselves into extraordinary attitudes, with much stuttering and stammering, they recounted the great deeds they had done in war, and the others all chimed in with great "Hoos" and "Hoofs" of approval, stamping on the ground like angry bulls. Some of these men fought against us in the Zulu War. After the dance was over, one very line fellow was introduced to us as the man who had carried a lot of Englishmen out of the mine when it was on fire a year or two ago.

I think it is a wonderful system by which all these tribes—that have hated each other for generations—can be made to live together in one compound, working side by side, and earning very good wages. They have separate huts and messes, but they buy at the same store, and share the same chapel, hospital, and swimming-bath.

There are about 2000 men in the compound, and they all seemed very happy. No beer or spirits are allowed. Any man who likes can learn to read and write while he is in the compound; and many of them were sitting round the fires, where they were boiling their mealy meal, reading to their mates.

We went into the hospital, which was very clean and trim. Natives in white suits, acting as attendants, showed us with pride their neatly-kept charts. There were one or two minor accidents in, and some bad cases of pneumonia, but they all appeared well cared for and comfortable.

The lady who lent me her horse has now returned to Kimberley, so I have not had so much riding lately; but the other night we had a glorious scamper out to Alexanderfontein by moonlight. About ten of us went, and we had supper out there. We had rather a mixed lot of horses and saddlery, and on the way back first one saddle came to grief, and then another. I distributed my gear by degrees—a girth to a gentleman who was riding with only one girth and it gave way, and I had two; a stirrup to a lady who dropped hers, and came off in consequence; and one of my reins to another lady, whose horse was too excited by the crowd of us, and required to be led. The others chaffed me, and begged for the bridle, and then for the saddle!

Now I am busy packing up for home, and trying to arrange things for my brother, who, when I go, intends to move into a smaller house just opposite to the club. There is also a good deal of tennis on just now, and between whiles I am struggling to pay my farewell calls. I was rather surprised to find there were about forty people I ought to call on; and as Kimberley does not wake up from its siesta until 4 P.M., and it is dark by 6 P.M. now, it is difficult to get through things, and George will have to take some P.P.C. cards round for me.

R.M.S. "SCOT," BAY OF BISCAY,
July 1893.

I am sorry I neglected to post this yarn from Kimberley; but I believe I will still post it when I land, as I may not see you yet awhile, and it will bring the history of my travels up to date.

I was more sorry to leave Kimberley than I expected to be; but I suppose one can't live in a place for a year without making some friends whom you are sorry to leave.

I journeyed down to the Cape all alone; but some Cape Town friends came to see me off, and it was quite home-like to be on the *Scot* once more.

The chief officer invited me to sit at his table, and we have had a delightful voyage, good weather, and pleasant people.

We had a few hours ashore at Madeira, and I think the flowers seem more beautiful every time I go there. Some day I should like to stay some weeks in the island.

We were all shocked to hear of the wreck of the *Victoria* off Tripoli, and the loss of 420 lives; it does seem terrible.

We find that, if all goes well, we should land on the day of the wedding of the Duke of York and Princess May.

The Bay of Biscay is behaving like a lamb. This is the fourth time I have been through it, and only once has it kicked up its heels and been really disagreeable.

I am going to spend a few days in town before I go home, so as to be interviewed by two or three matrons of the big hospitals. I think I know which hospital I would like best to get into, but whether I can persuade that particular matron that she really will have a vacancy in the autumn (I must spend a little time at home first), and that I really am the most suitable candidate for that particular vacancy, remains to be proved.

I am rather thin in consequence of the heat, but I am as brown as a berry; so I am sure they ought to think I look tough enough for the work.

XII

It is a long time since I last wrote to you, but there has not been much of interest to write about.

I tried very hard to get into some London hospital last autumn, but could not find a vacancy in any really good one, so I made up my mind it was better to wait for a vacancy here—where I had always wanted to train—than to slip in anywhere, where I did not *know* that the training was good. So I have just stayed at home, and in the summer played tennis and cricket, and learnt to make butter and jam, &c., and in the winter had a little hunting (on rather a stupid horse that was always doing something foolish, and one day distinguished himself by lying down at the meet!), and helped to teach in the night-school, where big lads and men, who had been cutting turnips for the sheep all day, came in the evenings to learn arithmetic, geography, &c., with much perseverance.

I went to help at the N. General Hospital for a month in the autumn, as they had a lot of nurses ill. It was rather funny, as I was sent to a men's ward (35 beds) as staff nurse; and of course I had had to do only with children before, so I had to pretend to know rather more than I did.

I had been there only a few days when the Sister of my ward went off duty with influenza, and there did not seem to be any one to come in her place; so we had to muddle along without a Sister. But everything went on all right, and the patients did well.

The Matron asked me to stay on permanently; but I thought a London certificate would be more valuable afterwards, so I only stayed until their sick nurses were able to return to duty.

I rather enjoyed my time there. The rough cleaning work that we had had to do at the Children's Hospital was all done by ward-maids, so we were able to give all our attention to the actual nursing; also our food was better, and more plentiful. But in spite of these things, there seemed to be a great deal of grumbling amongst the nurses. I was not accustomed to this, and I was not there long enough to learn whether they really had any good cause for their complaints.

The work was certainly hard, but that was partly because so many sisters and nurses were off duty ill; and when the doctors found that I was doing the Sister's work as well as my own, they were most considerate in trying to save me trouble.

I had been promised a vacancy here "in the summer" as an ordinary probationer for three years' training. Then, one day early in February, I had a wire from the Matron asking me whether I would like to enter as a lady pupil "if my fees were arranged for," and if so, I was to go up to see her the next day. I could not understand a bit what it meant, but thought I had better investigate. So up I trotted to town, and the Matron explained to me that they have a system here of working in two ranks, officers and privates. The officers are the sisters, and they are recruited from the lady pupils; the privates are the probationers, who might rise to be staff nurses, but beyond that there is no promotion from the ranks. Therefore, if I entered as a probationer, as I had arranged, I could never rise to be a sister.

Then she told me that it was probable there would be two or three vacancies for sisters in about a year, and a lady who was interested in the hospital had offered to pay the fees for some lady pupil, who would otherwise have entered as a probationer, so that she might have the advantage of the chance of promotion; and the Matron had decided to give me the offer, partly on account of my having had previous training. Of course there is no *promise* of promotion, as that must depend on one's work; but there is the chance of it. Did you ever hear of such good luck?

Of course I was only too glad to accept, and they wanted me at once; so I had to get my kit ready in a hurry, and began work here in February.

This is a huge place, quite a little town in itself, and I am very happy here.

I think I have been lucky in being first sent to a men's medical ward of forty beds. The Sister is a first-rate nurse and a splendid manager. She works hard herself, and expects every one else to do the same; so the ward always looks trim, and the patients are very comfortable.

My short experience at N. has been very useful to me, and I don't feel so much at sea in doing things for the men.

I find that, as lady pupil, I am really acting as "sister's assistant." I go round with Sister with the doctors, and if she is engaged with one doctor and another one comes, I have to escort him round; and it is necessary for me to know all about the cases, so as to be able to report about them. Another of my duties is to give all the medicines, and that for forty medical cases takes up a good deal of time. I also have charge of four beds, and do everything for the patients in them.

There are two staff nurses and two probationers (also two ward-maids), and I fill in my spare time with helping them in bed-making, carrying round meals, &c.; but I don't seem to be expected to do any of the cleaning work, and if I am busy helping Sister, the routine work goes on just the same without my assistance. I am not quite sure that it is a good arrangement, as one of the staff nurses in this ward has been here for years and years, and the other one for over three years, so of course they know more about the cases than I do; and I should think a brand new lady pupil, who had had no training before, might find it rather difficult. But I must say the staffs have been very nice to me. I didn't mean to let it be known that I "had been out before," but it leaked out.

There are about twenty of us lady pupils, and we live in the Matron's house. We have all our meals in the large nurses' dining-hall—but at a separate table—except supper, which we have in the sisters' dining-hall. The food is ever so much better than it was at the Children's Hospital. Some of the nurses grumble at it; but I think wherever people feed in a crowd there are always some who grumble. At any rate, it is not *necessary* to buy food here.

At first I had rather uninteresting cases in my beds, but now Sister is giving me some good ones. I have one jolly fat baby of two and a half with tonsilitis, who was sent to us from a women's ward, because they were not sure that he was not going in for diphtheria, and they had other children in the ward. I had to do a good deal of treatment for him at first, and he hated it; but now he has forgiven me, and we are excellent friends, and all the men are doing their best to spoil him.

Then I have a poor man with Bright's disease, who is very ill. He is a curious-looking object, as he is quite bald, and he likes to wear a red knitted cap in bed. He is often delirious now in the evenings, and then he uses very bad language. When Sister is out in the evening, I have to read prayers in the ward. At first I was very shy of reading before all these men, especially when some of them are of quite a superior class; and when I was in the middle of prayers the other evening, my bald-headed man chimed in with a lot of bad language. It was really very trying, and I knew if either of the nurses went to remonstrate with him, he would only continue in a louder voice; so I had to shorten the prayers somewhat. If he continues like this, I am afraid he will have to go to the strong-room; but up there they have only male attendants, and we are rather loth to send him off, as he is really very ill, and needs a lot of nursing.

A sad thing happened the other day. We had an old man in very ill with angina pectoris; he had great difficulty in breathing, and could not lie down at all. I was always trying to prop him up and make him comfortable. He got very little rest, but he was always so good and grateful. He was not one of my own cases; but he was on several medicines (to be given as required), so I had to go to him very often for one thing and another. One day I was going round giving the two o'clock medicines, and when I got to his bed, he was lying back on his pillows apparently asleep. It was so unusual for him to look at all comfortable, I thought I would certainly not disturb him for his medicine. Sister was talking to a doctor a few yards away, and I was just going to point out to her that the old man was resting, when something made me turn back and look at him more closely, and I found he was quite dead. Poor old fellow, he was indeed "resting." I just pulled a screen round him, and then called Sister and the house surgeon; but he was quite gone, and even the man in the next bed had not noticed any change.

XIII

With much sorrow I left my nice and interesting men's medical ward, and found myself landed in a smaller surgical and accident ward for women and children. There could hardly have been a greater contrast. There everything was done with order and method, and well done; here every one seems to rush about in a breathless way, and the ward never looks tidy, and I am quite sure that the bustle that goes on is bad for the serious cases.

I am responsible for eight cases instead of four, and at first I thought I should never get them all washed in time in the morning; but now I find so many of them can do a good deal more for themselves than the medical cases could; also the medicines in a surgical ward are nothing to those in a medical; so I get through all right, and keep up to time.

Three surgeons have beds in the ward, and that makes the work a little difficult, as sometimes they all arrive at the same time, and sometimes they all want to operate at the same time. This is most awkward, as we have not got fittings for them all, and have to run backwards and forwards for things. They seem to me a most amiable set of surgeons; I know the surgeons at our Children's Hospital would not have put up with being kept waiting as these men do; but I do hate not having everything they want ready before they ask for it. However, I am beginning to feel my way, and I think I shall soon be able to get different sets of things ready to use in these emergencies.

It took me some time to find out why the ward was always in a state of chaos, and it is only because you are so far away that I can safely tell you the reason. I believe it is simply and solely because the Sister, though a fairly good nurse, is really no good as a Sister. I am sorry to say it, as she has been very nice to me, and the poor thing tries her best. She runs about, and does many things that the junior probationers ought to do, but she has no idea of looking after the nurses; and as the staff nurse is rather a shirker, and is very fond of chattering to the dressers, the probationers who are keen to work are rather overworked, and those who are not keen don't work. Also, if there is a rush of work, Sister rather loses her head, and runs about in an aimless sort of way; and in the theatre, if anything goes wrong, and they want things in a hurry, she always seems to hand the wrong thing.

I find it a bit difficult, as the doctors get in the way of turning to me if they want things quickly. As soon as I found out what was wrong with the ward, and that Sister was quite nice and "meant well," but just had not got it in her to be a good manager, I made up my mind that the ward *should* be a smart ward, in spite of obstacles, and really it is improving by degrees.

I have been having a good deal of correspondence lately about a small boy who, Sister said, would have to go to the workhouse when he leaves here, and I thought he was a suitable case for Dr. Barnardo's Homes; so she said I could try if I could get him in there, and I have just succeeded in doing so.

His mother died when he was born, and his father appears to be a thoroughly bad lot, generally in prison. This boy had lived with his old grandmother and run wild; a pretty little chap, but quite a heathen, and fond of using bad language in the most innocent way. He came in here for a small operation, and while he has been here his grandmother died very suddenly. The people at Dr. Barnardo's Homes have been very good about it, made all inquiries for themselves, and got the father's consent. Now they have agreed to take him as soon as he is well. He is a plucky little chap, and I suppose they will probably ship him over to Canada one day, and that will give him a better start in life than he might get from a workhouse.

I think we get very good times off duty here—one hour off one day, and three hours off the next; and the sisters and lady pupils have a Saturday to Monday once a month—that means from 4 P.M. on Saturday to 10 A.M. on Monday.

When I was moved to this ward, I just missed my Saturday to Monday; so, to make up for it, they gave me "extra leave" last week from Saturday afternoon to Monday night, and it just happened to be May week at Cambridge, so I went down and had such a jolly time. B. seems to be very happy at Clare, and to have very nice friends there. My sister was up for all the week, and having a first-rate time, going to all the dances, &c. It was my first visit to Cambridge, and there was so much to see. It ought to be easy to work when you are in such beautiful surroundings.

On the way back the engine of my train broke down, and I did not get in till 11 P.M., and I had to go and confess the next morning in the office that I was late; but it was the first time I had been late since I came, so I was forgiven.

We had rather an exciting "take-in" week a fortnight or so ago: first of all a poor, tiny baby with a very badly-cut throat (done by its mother, who had afterwards proceeded to cut her own throat, and killed herself). They did tracheotomy for the baby, but it lived only a few hours. Then came a poor little girl of eight, very badly burnt. She had had to get up to light the fire while her mother lay in bed (from her looks, I should think the mother had been drinking), and the child managed to set herself on fire. I think she will pull round, but it will be a long time before she will be able to walk again. She does not have much pain now, and I think she is quite enjoying herself here. The next case was another cut throat—a poor, feeble-looking woman, whose husband had first cut her throat and then his own. He is in the male accident ward, and not very much damaged; she is a good deal damaged, but I think they will both recover.

I had arranged to go to the Academy with L., as it was my free afternoon; but this poor woman came in soon after dinner, and I knew she would have to go up to the theatre, so I wired to L. that I could not meet her. And it was just as well I did, as three more accidents came in that afternoon, and one of these too had to go to the theatre (a compound fracture of the tibia and fibula); so we had a rushing time.

Yesterday was theatre day for our ward; and as Sister had had to retire to bed with a sick-headache, I had the honour of taking our cases up to the theatre. I was rather nervous, as it was the first time I had been up alone for our senior surgeon, and he had one bad case—an excision of knee. But the other three cases were not very bad ones, and we got along all right.

For the last three months we have been having a very interesting course of lectures on physiology, and the girl who shares my room and I spend all our spare minutes in reading up the subject. She is clever, but has not read much physiology before, so I have been able to help her a bit; and I should not be surprised if she does better in the exam. than I do. We are both of us looked upon as quite juniors amongst the lady pupils; but I don't fancy the seniors are taking much trouble, beyond just writing out their notes of the lectures, so I hope we shall do pretty decently. It is not easy to get much time to read when you have a heavy ward to wrestle with; but I am sure it helps you in exams. if you can manage to read rather more than you are absolutely obliged to about what the lecturer is trying to stuff into you in a condensed form.

I have been here six months now, and may get sent off for my holiday any day; but there has been some delay on account of Sister not being very well. She does not seem to want me to leave, as I shall probably not get sent back to this ward afterwards; but it has been very hot of late, and I shall be glad of a rest.

XIV

After my last letter to you I was bundled off for my holiday. I was glad enough to get it, but I missed the last two physiology lectures. This was rather a bore, as the exam. was the day after I got back; so I had no chance of borrowing any one's notes of those lectures, as I was supposed to do. However, I came out third, and my stable companion was first amongst the lady pupils—not so bad for two juniors; and we heard that four or five of the seniors had a little interview with the Matron in her office, and were advised to work rather harder before the next exam.

Now we are having lectures on dispensing, and they are the most interesting lectures I have struck yet. We go down to the dispensary, and the head-dispenser makes us mess about, and make up prescriptions, and make pills, powders, &c. We fire off questions at each other at odd moments, when we meet—and also in bed at night—as to the various doses of different drugs, and what they are prescribed for, and the antidotes for different poisons, &c.

I was sent to a very nice women's medical ward on my return from my holiday, and had some interesting work there. The Sister was very nice to me (she has been here for years, and many of the lady pupils don't like her, but she is a first-rate nurse), and she gave me very good cases. One of my first cases was a little girl of ten with typhoid fever. She was very ill for some weeks, and then such a poor little wasted skeleton of a child! It was very nice feeding her up, when once it was safe to do so; and her great big eyes used to follow me about the ward, wondering what the next feed was going to be.

Sister said that I could hardly have had a more instructive case, as she had nearly all the bad symptoms a typhoid case can have, including a good deal of hæmorrhage.

I was horribly proud one day when the senior physician was going round and lecturing to the students and speaking to them of the necessity for good nursing in typhoid; and he made Sister show them the child's poor, bony little back and legs, with not a red mark on them; and he told them it had taken all her strength to battle with the fever, and if she had also had a bed-sore to sap her strength away, she could never have pulled through.

We had two diphtheria tracheotomies while I was in that ward; and though they were not my cases (as they both had special nurses), I was present at the operations, and I learnt a good deal about their treatment, as Sister used to let me relieve their nurses for meals, &c. And she taught me to change and clean their tubes, and so on; so that when I was put on as a special later on, I was not so much afraid of accidents as I should otherwise have been.

It must have been a very bad form of diphtheria, as one of the specials became infected, and had to go away to the Fever Hospital; and then Sister took it, but she was not very ill with it, and she was nursed in her own room. It has made them talk about the necessity for some isolation ward to put these cases in. Of course they are only taken in here if they are too ill for it to be safe to send them on to the Fever Hospitals.

We had a busy time when Sister was ill, but the staff nurse was very good and to be depended upon, and things went on all right.

I must tell you of a little joke we had one night in the Matron's house, where all the lady pupils live. Late one evening in September, when we were all undressed, one of them came to my room and said there was a wretched cat on some leads outside the bathroom window, and it was making such a row, as it could not escape. We went to inspect, and agreed that a rescue was necessary. By this time most of the lady pupils had assembled, and we fetched a ladder from the boxroom. It was too short; but we tied bath towels to it, and lowered it through the window to the leads. Then the stupid cat would not come up, and only cried the more; so I was shoved through the window in my dressing-gown, and they held on to me until I got my feet on the ladder, and could climb down to the cat. Just then Matron's door opened, and they all slipped away to their rooms. I heard something about "too much noise" and "lights out," and then she came into the bathroom and shut down the window. It was lucky the ladder *was* too short, or she must have seen it. It was pretty dark, and I was sitting down consoling the cat and waiting till the coast was clear, when I heard a smothered laugh, and then for the first time I remembered the gardens at the back, that belonged to some of our visiting doctors. I had looked at their houses and seen all the blinds down, and I had never thought they might be sitting under the trees at that time of night. After that, I very carefully kept my face to the wall; and soon the window was cautiously opened, and with some difficulty the cat and I were hauled in, and very quietly we pulled up the ladder. Then I told them I was certain we had been watched, and we located the garden from which the laugh had come; and next morning, sure enough, there were two basket-chairs under the trees, so we knew which doctor it was. But he never gave us away, and I don't know to this day whether he recognised me; but I often fancied there was a twinkle in his eye when we met.

Then the question arose what to do with the cat, as it appeared to be hungry, and not inclined to be quiet; so eventually the most innocent-looking lady pupil was deputed to go to the home sister, and tell her she had caught this strange cat in the bathroom, and, as it seemed starving, might she go down and feed it, and then turn it out? The home sister was fond of cats, and her sympathies were aroused; so she assisted in providing it with supper and seeing it off the premises.

In November I was sent on night duty. The lady pupils are not obliged to do night duty, as they are only here for one year; but Matron was short of senior probationers, and asked me if I would like it, and I thought I would. Part of the time I have been an "extra," just helping wherever they were busy, and helping in the theatre for any night operations. Then I was put on as "special" with a tracheotomy (diphtheria) in a men's medical ward—such a nice boy, called Albert, aged eight. And, when he was getting better, another little chap of three came in, so desperately bad that they had to do tracheotomy in the receiving room; and then he was brought over and put in a cot by my boy's bed, and I looked after them both. Poor Albert was rather jealous at first, and whenever I was attending to the small boy he began to "wheeze" too, thinking I should rush to his rescue; but he soon found that that did not pay.

After these boys had both recovered, I disinfected, and had a night off to air myself; and then Matron let me do the staff nurse's nights off—very interesting, but rather anxious, work.

You go to a ward which perhaps you have never been inside before, and you don't know where anything is kept. There are from twenty to forty patients; if the latter, there is a probationer to help you. Most of them are sleeping quietly; the few who are awake are probably wondering what sort of a rise they can take out of the strange nurse.

Some of the sisters are very good about giving one a full written report; but other sisters are rather casual, telling you much of what you may or may not do for number eight or number eleven, but seeming impatient if you try to jot down notes.

The first night off I took was in a men's surgical ward, where there was a nice lad of eighteen who had had his leg amputated that day (for a tubercular knee). He was so good and patient, but of course he needed a good deal of attention, and I wished I could stay with him all the time; but there was an old man at the other end of the ward rather delirious, and he would insist upon saying his prayers with a loud voice, and confessing his sins to me, calling me "Maria, dear." I was thankful when the house surgeon came round and ordered him a sleeping-draught; but it took me quite half an hour to persuade him to drink it, and then it was a long time before it had any effect.

In another ward the sister told me that the patients needed nothing to be done for them until I gave them their breakfast in the morning, but "*would* I take great care of her Persian and Manx cats, and not let them escape from the ward?"

It was also airing night, so I had plenty to do airing sheets, &c., and putting on clean sheets in the morning; but it was not exciting.

To-night I am staff nurse in the men's accident ward; but there is a bright little pro. on as well, and she seems to be accustomed to do most of the work. We have had one case in—a van-boy with slight concussion of the brain; but I have got him washed, and he is now asleep with an ice-bag on his head. There are several bad cases in the ward, but they all seem inclined to sleep; so I am actually sitting down to finish up this scribble to you.

I like night duty; you seem to have more time to fad over the patients who are really bad, and to do little things for their comfort; and the convalescent ones generally sleep and don't worry you; but it is hard work sometimes, especially between 5 and 8 A.M., when every one wakes up, and every one wants something, and there are all the breakfasts to give round, and all the beds to make, and the temperatures to take, and the fomentations to change, and a hundred different things all needing to be done at once; and you rush around and expect every minute the day nurses will come in and say "What a muddle the ward is in!" and sometimes, when you are beautifully forward with your work and think Sister will be pleased, a house surgeon runs up in his pyjamas and dressing-gown to say he is sending in a bad case, and then you have to give all your attention to that case, and can't do the final clearing up for which you thought there would be heaps of time!

XV

GENERAL HOSPITAL, LONDON,
June 1895.

Many and various are the jobs I have done since my last letter, and now I must tell you that I am a full-blown Sister or, as they say here, I have got "my blue"; but I had better begin where I left off.

I was then bustling about on night duty, and I spent a very happy Christmas like that. Of course, we should all like to be at home for Christmas, but in hospital so much is done to make it bright and cheery for the patients, and so many of them have so little brightness in their lives, that it is nice to see how thoroughly they enjoy it.

They all have really nice presents; there is any amount of good food provided; plenty of entertainments (music, Christmas trees, &c.); and the men are allowed to smoke in the wards.

The doctors and students are really splendid in the way they work at decorating the wards, &c., and carrying the patients who are well enough about to other wards for entertainments.

The children of the slums around here will do anything to get into the hospital for Christmas, and the front surgery is full of little imps who have all got a "very bad pain!"

In January I had to retire to bed for a few days with a high temperature and a touch of influenza, and while I was in bed the day came for the dispensing exam., so I begged to be allowed to go, and vowed I was quite recovered, and they let me attend.

I made up my prescriptions (a bottle of medicine and some powders), and then I got under way with the paper, and thought it was rather a nice one, but before I reached the end my head began to swim, and I felt convinced I had mixed everything up and given all the wrong doses, and I thought what an ass I had been to try it, and I was certain I should come out at the bottom of the list!

One of my friends escorted me back to bed and took my temperature, and when she found it was 103 she went off and told the Matron; so next morning the doctor appeared, and I was kept in bed for a whole week, and then sent away for a few days' change, but before I went away Matron came to tell me that I was first in the dispensing exam., with 114 marks out of a possible 125. If I had any more exams. to go in for, I think I ought to arrange to have a little influenza beforehand, as it seems to stimulate my brain; but, thank goodness, that is my last.

You know I have always vowed that nothing would induce me to be a matron? Well, I have been rather near it; I have been acting as assistant matron for some time. First of all, the assistant matron was ill, and went away for a bit, and I did her work; then, when she came back, Matron went away for a fortnight, and I stayed on in the office helping the assistant.

It was rather interesting learning the ins and outs of the "Administrative Department," but I am still convinced that it is no catch to be a matron.

Sisters come to complain of a nurse, and you have to send for that nurse and scold her for her reported misdeeds, when, perhaps, all the time you have rather a feeling that Sister has been unreasonable in what she has expected of the girl.

Then nurses have a way of sometimes getting ill, and it always seems to be the nurse whose place it is most difficult to fill; then Matron goes out for the afternoon, saying to the assistant, "There are three extra nurses, and I have sent them to Wards A., B., and C., where they are busy, so no one is likely to ask you for another extra," and as soon as she has gone a house surgeon runs in to say he has sent in a very bad diphtheria case to Ward D. for immediate tracheotomy, and can I send specials over at once? I look on the list to see who the three extras are, and find not one of them is suitable to take on the case—one is going for her holiday in a few days and the other two are quite juniors—so I rack my brain to think which of the ward nurses is most suitable, and fix upon Pro. 1 in Ward A., as she has nursed one or two tracheotomies; so I have to interview Sister A., and she is most reluctant to give up her Pro. 1, and is quite certain Matron would not have taken her away, but I have to be firm and try to console her by sending her the best extra in place of Pro. 1 (thereby incurring black looks from Sister B., who is quite sure her ward is far heavier than Sister A.'s!); some one ought to be sent to bed to be ready to act as night special, but I conclude that can wait till Matron returns, as she may have some nurse she has promised to put on as special. That is the sort of work the assistant matron has to do—a good deal of fagging about and acting as a sort of buffer between the sisters and the Matron, much writing of letters and other work in the office, and a good deal of carving at meal times—one Sunday I carved roast beef for seventy nurses, some of them day nurses and some of them night.

I had just come to the end of my time in the office (I was still a lady pupil then), when an appeal came to the Matron to lend two staff nurses to one of the large London Infirmaries, where they had a great many nurses ill.

I volunteered to go (as I thought it would be a new experience), and then another lady pupil also volunteered.

It was a pouring wet evening in March when we set off in a hansom cab, the other lady pupils rather jeering at us, and saying that when *they* went to the workhouse they should do the thing correctly in an aged four-wheeler!

We had no idea where the Infirmary was, but trusted to the cabby, and after a long drive he turned into a stone-paved yard and drew up at a heavily-barred door; it looked more like a prison than an infirmary, but I got out in the rain to explore, and after a little while I managed to explain to the old man in charge that I did not wish to apply for admission to the Casual Ward, but to find the Infirmary. He told me that was more than a mile farther on; so the weary horse plodded on once more, and eventually brought us to an imposing building, where, in three weeks of hard work, we learnt many things.

They were very busy and very short-handed. I was sent to a women's medical ward of thirty-two beds, but the place was so full that I had thirty-six patients, the extra ones sleeping on mattresses on the floor. For the first week, whenever a patient came in, I had to consider which of those in beds was the most capable of turning out and descending to the floor, to make room for the new-comer, but after that things quieted down, and before I left the patients were reduced to the correct number.

There was a sister in charge of my ward and of another one just opposite of the same size. For a few days I worked with the staff nurse, and then she had to leave, and I was left to do the work of the ward with the help of a probationer, who came in for an hour and a half every morning, and who relieved me when I went off duty every other day; and on the alternate days, when the staff nurse from the opposite ward was off duty, I had to patrol her ward at intervals, and give the probationer any help she needed.

At first I was appalled at the small number of the nursing staff for so many beds, but I soon found that everything was done in a way very different from our hospital methods, and that if we worked hard and fast it was possible to do all that was really necessary for the patients, but quite impossible to do the little faddy things that make so much difference to their comfort.

For one thing, the convalescent patients were expected to do a great deal of the routine ward work, and, as a rule, the convalescents stayed in much longer than they do in a hospital, so they were more fit to assist, but this hardly applied to my short time in the Infirmary, owing to the great pressure on the beds; also I found that there were only about six or eight out of the thirty-six patients really acutely ill, so I was able to give most of my attention to them—three of them were absolutely helpless, and needed much care and nursing.

The rest of them were chiefly old ladies who were just not strong enough for the workhouse life, and so were drafted into the Infirmary; most of them were able to get out of bed and potter about the ward. This they loved to do with very scanty clothing on—rather to my horror—and I found that when a doctor was sighted on his way to the ward it was best to clap my hands vigorously, when all the old dames scuttled into bed like so many rabbits into their holes.

Poor old things, several of them had evidently seen better days, and there were many sad stories to be listened to, and they did so much appreciate the little I could do for their comfort.

It was very hard work, as one always seemed to be working against time, but I quite enjoyed my three weeks in the Infirmary. Matron had not told us we were to be paid for this work, so when we each received £6. 6s. for the three weeks, we felt very rich!

We were quite glad to return to our good old hospital, and since then I have been doing Sister's holiday work, and now I have just been appointed Sister in the front surgery (where all the new cases and accidents come in); it is utterly different from being in the wards, but I think I shall find it interesting—at any rate for a time. I shall wait to tell you about it until I have been here a little longer, and have taken my bearings more correctly.

XVI

General Hospital, London,
January 1896.

I think I shall be rather glad when I get a ward of my own and settle down; but every one seems to think I am lucky in getting such varied experience, so I suppose I ought to be grateful, and it is not yet two years since I first entered here.

I spent six months as Sister in the front surgery, and it was very interesting.

There had never been a sister in charge there before, but just one old staff nurse, who had let the dressers do just what they liked, and there was a lot of waste and much disorder.

Matron gave me a very good probationer, and she was just as keen on getting the place nice and trim as I was. It took us a week or two to get all the drawers &c., scrubbed out and tidy, and a good many more weeks before we got all the splints sorted and padded.

The Medical Superintendent was pleased, because I managed to reduce the cost of dressings every week from £10 to £7 before I had been there a month, and it was still further reduced after a few more weeks.

Of course it is difficult for young dressers (who come on for only three months at a time) to understand how much difference a little extravagance in each dressing makes in the weekly bills; and they can't be expected to know the relative value of different kinds of wool, &c., unless it is pointed out to them, but as a rule, when they do understand, they are quite willing to use the cheaper dressings (for cases where they do just as well) provided that we keep a supply ready to their hands.

I often wonder whether, when people go round a hospital and see the rows of white beds and clean patients, and everything neat and tidy, they think the patients arrive here looking like that. Very often in the wards, when the porters have carried up an accident case on the stretcher, I have hardly known how to get the man's dirty clothes off, and it takes time before you can get them reasonably clean; but in the wards you always receive a note or a message by the porter from the house surgeon, with a rough diagnosis of what the case is, so that you know which limb to be especially careful in moving. But it is different when you receive a patient in the front surgery; the policemen tramp in and deposit the stretcher on the floor, and there is much mopping of their foreheads before they tell you roughly what they know of the accident, and then you have to proceed to find out for yourself what is the extent of the injury, and often the patient is quite unconscious, so he cannot help you at all.

I think at first I had a dim notion that every case that was carried in on a stretcher was sure to be admitted to the wards, but one soon learns that a good many of these cases are more frightened than hurt, and after a little rest and a thorough overhaul by the house surgeon they are able to go home again; on the other hand, every now and then a man who has had a very serious accident will manage to walk up to the hospital, and he may even sit down amongst the other waiting patients and quietly wait his turn to be seen, unless you happen to be on the look-out, and note that he is looking ill, and get him on to a couch for immediate attention.

There is generally plenty doing in the front surgery, and whenever any of the men have nothing better to do they stroll in to see what is going on, so one hears all the gossip of the place; very quaint, too, are the tales the patients tell of their symptoms. I am not good at remembering these things, but there was one old lady who said the doctor told her that she had "the brownkitis, and that all her tubs (tubes) were full up."

Sometimes we had exciting times. I remember one morning when I came on duty the night nurse reported that a bad case of compound fracture of the jaw and other injuries had come in, and been taken straight up to the theatre, and that the house surgeon and all the available dressers were busy with it then. She had no sooner gone away than in tramped four big policemen with a stretcher, which they deposited on the floor; on uncovering the patient I found a poor man on whose head several heavy planks had fallen. Part of the scalp was torn up, and it was bleeding profusely. I sent my probationer flying to the theatre to ask for some one to come to help, and then I made one policeman put pressure with his finger on an artery on one side of the head and another policeman on the other, while I collected some dressings, forceps, &c. Much to my astonishment, first one policeman fainted and subsided on the floor, and then the other one did the same (the other two had gone outside); then the probationer returned to say the man in the theatre was bad, and they could not spare any one, but some one would come as soon as possible. Just then the police inspector walked in, and his look of astonishment at his two prostrate men was very fine, but he called the other two men to move them, and then he gave me the help I needed, while the probationer and I did what we could to stop the hæmorrhage; it was pretty well subdued by the time the house surgeon got down, but he saw at once it was a bad case, and took the man straight up to the theatre. As soon as he had gone we dosed the two policemen with Mist. Ammonia, but it was a little while before they were fit to return to duty, and then we were just thinking we would begin our much delayed morning's work when, strangely enough, two men were carried in dead, the two stretchers arriving within a few minutes of each other; one was a suicide from the Thames, and the dressers tried artificial respiration for some time, but the poor chap was quite dead; the other was a poor old gentleman who had apparently died of heart failure when hurrying to catch a train.

We saw a great many infectious diseases in the front surgery, and had to keep them in an isolation room till the fever ambulance came to fetch them. I remember one day when we had samples of nearly all the infectious fevers to despatch—first came a case of smallpox, then one of scarlet fever, then one of diphtheria, and there were also cases of measles and chickenpox, but these had to be sent back to their homes. There was quite an outbreak of smallpox just then (I think we had twenty cases in the front surgery in one week), so everybody in the hospital who had not been recently vaccinated had to be done, and we were all very sorry for ourselves for a time.

Another little episode in the front surgery was when a baby took us all by surprise by being born there! We should have sent it on to the Infirmary, but the mother was rather bad, so we had to take them in.

One Sunday evening I was in chapel when I heard some one come to the door, and then the porter came to fetch me, and at the door I found one of the dressers who told me there was a bad compound fracture in the surgery, and the house surgeon would be glad if I would come, as he wanted to give an anæsthetic. When I got there I found a crowd of men all standing round a poor little dog with a badly crushed leg! so we got some suitable splints, and they gave it an anæsthetic and put up the fracture; then they sent word to the male accident ward to get a fracture bed ready for a patient, and the porters were secured to carry it along on a big stretcher. It was in the hospital for some weeks, and got quite well again.

Just before Christmas the Matron was obliged to go home for a time, so once more I was asked to go on duty as assistant matron. Christmas is always a busy time all over the hospital, and in the office (with the Matron away) we had more than enough to do—so many presents to receive and acknowledge and distribute, and many visitors to show round, &c. Then, after Christmas, a good many nurses got ill (some with influenza), and every one seemed to be wanting special nurses at the same time, and all were quite hurt that I could not make new nurses to order.

So I was not sorry when the sister of the nicest ward in the hospital told me that she had been appointed Matron of another hospital (she had been here for years), and as she knew nothing of office work she wanted to ask Matron if she would have her in the office for a few weeks' experience. I thought it would mean that I should go back to the front surgery, and I was quite pleased, but instead of that, Matron wrote to ask me to take over that sister's ward for a couple of months, as she had not got a suitable sister ready to take it permanently (it is always given to one of the seniors here); so I was still more pleased, especially when I found that the pay was at the rate of £10 a year more than for the other wards.

This is an awfully nice ward of thirty-two beds, in two divisions—one for men, and one for women and children. It is chiefly for medical cases, but there is a small theatre attached, and a good many abdominal operations are done; there is also a private ward, to which the surgeons can send any operation cases that need especial attention; and they have special nurses.

In the wards I have a good staff, as it is always considered the most acute ward in the hospital, and I can generally get an extra nurse if I want, so I don't do much actual nursing myself, but there seem to be doctors constantly going round whom I have to attend, and somehow I always seem to be busy.

The longer I am in hospital the more I see how much harder it is to be responsible for other people's work than just for your own, and I can quite understand why so many of the staff nurses much prefer to do all the best part of the nursing themselves than to teach the probationers and let them do it; but it is a wrong principle, as the probationers must be taught, and we must learn to trust others (even when we know we could do things quicker and better ourselves), and to increase the trust just in proportion as we find them worthy of it; that is where the art of the teacher comes in!

XVII

I think I last wrote when I had just taken charge of C. Ward for two months.

I had a most interesting time there, and was quite sorry to give it up, but it was hard work. Unlike the other wards, that "take in" new cases for a week and then have a rest, C. is always "taking in," as the men in charge see every new case that comes up to the hospital (except accidents), and they can take them in if they like, as long as there are any beds empty in the ward; and if they don't think it is a particularly interesting case, it is passed on to the house surgeons or house physicians for the other wards; but, of course, they try their best to get all the most interesting cases for themselves; consequently the sister is never free to go out with any confidence that no new cases can be landed in while she is away; and when you do go out you generally find on your return that something has happened that makes you wish you had never gone!

Still I learnt a great deal in my time in that ward, and I enjoyed it. The physicians' talks with the students over these "selected cases" were most instructive.

Soon after I took charge we had a run of tracheotomies; the first was a dear, fat baby of thirteen months, but it had diphtheria very badly, and was not a hopeful case from the first; not many hours after it was operated upon another came in—a sweet little boy of three called "Alex." He was much relieved by the operation, and got on so well; but the poor baby ran a temperature of 106° all through the second day, and died late that evening with a temperature of 108°, in spite of all we could do for it. I believe we were much more cut up about losing it than the mother was; she did not seem to mind a bit, and apparently had made all her plans for the funeral beforehand—and it was such a pretty baby too!

The special nurses I had for these tracheotomies had never nursed one before, so you can imagine I could not leave them alone much, and was thankful I had had a good many to nurse when I was a lady pupil.

We had one very curious case. A young man was brought in unconscious one afternoon about 2 P.M.; a little after five he got worse, and his respiration suddenly stopped, the pulse went on steadily, so they did artificial respiration; this went on till 9.30 P.M., and then they decided to trephine, thinking it must be a cerebral tumour pressing on the brain; of course no anæsthetic was necessary, as the poor man showed no sign of life except that the pulse was beating; they could not find any tumour, so he was put back to bed, and the men went on doing artificial respiration all through the night in turns, until the pulse suddenly stopped at 9.15 A.M., sixteen hours after the respiration had ceased—a very strange case.

We often had rushing days, when it seemed impossible to make time for meals, and scarcely time to breathe. I remember one day especially, when we took in seven new cases, two of them, curiously enough, men from quite different districts, who had both taken oxalic acid with a view to suicide; one was an old man who was very bad for a day or two, and then seemed to be getting better, but died suddenly one night from heart failure; and the other was a poor young fellow of thirty, who had been waiter in one shop for eight years, and was then turned off by a new manager and replaced by a German lad. He had a wretched wife who drank, and she took away his clothes and then disappeared; so we had to rig him up in a suit when he went off; one of the other patients gave me five shillings for him, and he asked me to keep it till he had been before the magistrates, as he thought he would be sent to prison, but he came back after his appearance in the police courts to tell me he had been let off with a caution, and he thought his old master would take him back; such a nice, quiet-mannered man, and most anxious to do anything to help the nurses in their work, or to wait on the other patients, and they all liked him.

The same day one of the house surgeons was admitted with a badly poisoned arm, and a friend of one of the students with typhoid fever; he had it very badly and caused us much anxiety, but pulled through all right in the end.

After this spell in C. Ward I expected to return to my front surgery, but instead I was offered in March (and gladly accepted) the post of Night Sister, and that is what I have been doing ever since, except for an interval for my summer holiday, and also for a few weeks when I took charge of a large male medical ward while the sister had her holiday.

Being Night Sister here means plenty of running about, and plenty of responsibility, but it also means better pay than Ward Sister, so that suited me all right.

They are talking of having two night sisters soon—one medical and one surgical—and there would be plenty of work for two, as we have a good deal of theatre work in the night, and sometimes I cannot help being worried when I am kept long in the theatre with urgent cases, and I know there are bad cases over in the medical buildings (sometimes with only rather junior nurses in charge of them), and I can't get round to visit them.

I have charge of about six hundred beds, and they are divided into twenty-one wards (of course nurses in each ward and two nurses in the large wards); I have to go all round three times every night, and run in much oftener to see any bad cases, and the nurses send for me in any difficulty; there is a slate in my office for messages, and when I return after my rounds I often find two or three messages, "Please come at once to P."; "Please come to N.—urgent," and so on, and I have to fly to whichever I think is likely to be the most urgent.

The morning round always takes the longest, as all the patients are then awake, and I have to say good morning to them all, and remember to ask after their particular aches and pains, and it is not very easy to remember what is the matter with them all, though I know very well all the details about those who are very ill and have much done for them in the night.

There is one place I don't enjoy visiting, and that is the strong room at the top of the surgical buildings. Lately we seem to have had so many men who go off their heads (generally from drink), and if they are left in the wards they disturb the other patients so much that it is better for them to be moved, and then they have male attendants up there; but these male attendants are not members of our regular staff (I wish they were), and I never feel that I quite know their capabilities, or how much I can trust them, and more than once I have found them asleep; so I have to go up very often when any patient is bad there.

I remember one night we had a very lively time of rushing about. We began with a man who had cut his throat—not very bad, but he had to go up to the theatre; then a lady who had taken three ounces of laudanum, and the doctors had to keep her walking up and down the corridor, with a weary porter on each side of her, for six hours before they thought it safe to let her turn into a bed; then I was called to a poor man in Ward P., who got worse, and died rather suddenly—a phthisis case; next a tracheotomy came in, and had to be done at once, and while we were all busy with it a baby was born in Ward D.; but the day sister had to be called to attend to that, as I was mixed up with the diphtheria case, and could not go near a confinement; then a fractured femur came in, and next an acute pneumonia—rather delirious. In the intervals of receiving these new cases and sorting them to the different wards we had to brew strong coffee and administer it to the lady who had taken poison, and provide refreshments for the porters who were minding her. In the early morning she was allowed to go to bed and to sleep; she recovered very soon, and I don't think she will do it again!

I joined the Royal National Pension Fund for Nurses a few months ago; it seems to be a good thing, and if I can only keep up the premiums I shall have the noble pension of about £20 or so when I am fifty; it will keep me in extras when I retire to the workhouse, as I am certain no one can go on nursing for a great many years at the pace we have to go in hospital.

Just now I am having a rest (and another sister is rushing about on night duty), as I have been warded for the past fortnight, and in a few days I hope to go home for a change.

I had a cold for many weeks, and did not pay much attention to it, as I thought it was only because I was about all night and did not get enough sunshine to help me to throw it off; but then I got very bad headaches, so I had to see a doctor, and he passed me on to our nose specialist, who has been most awfully kind, coming down every day, and sometimes twice a day, to see me. It was not really a cold, but some disease in the antrum, and he has done two small operations for me, and it has been horridly painful, but now it is getting well rapidly, and every one has been most awfully good to me, and I am beginning to feel less of a limp rag than I have done for some time past.

It was funny spending Christmas as a patient instead of running about looking after the patients; but it was nearly my first day up, so I was glad enough to be lazy, and I have had many visitors, so it has not been dull at all.

XVIII

GENERAL HOSPITAL, LONDON,
September 1897.

Just now I am feeling so sorrowful at the prospect of leaving this hospital (my home for the last three and a half years) that I hardly know how to give my attention to telling you how the last few months have been spent.

No, I have not been turned out, and they have given me a first-class certificate, and are good enough to say that they are very sorry I am going, and perhaps they will have me back again some day!

I think I was warded when I wrote to you last, and after that they sent me home for a little rest. Whenever I go home some one in the village gets ill, or some child gets scalded, or some accident happens; they seem to think it is necessary to keep my hand in; but during that visit home my only patient was poor Jessie, the family cat! It was Sunday evening, and we were all sitting in the dining-room just after prayers, when poor Jessie hobbled in, really screaming with pain. One leg had evidently been caught in a trap, and there was a bad compound fracture which she could not bear me to handle, so I said we must either have some chloroform or the poor dear must be shot. The nearest doctor (and chloroform) was three miles away, but C. volunteered to fetch some, and went off on his bicycle, while I prepared some splints and strapping, &c., and poor Jessie used bad language under the table.

I have sometimes had to hold an obstreperous child while it has been given chloroform, but that is nothing to holding a cat! However, at last we got her under, and then put the fracture in good position and stitched up the wound, securing the leg very firmly on splints; this operation was watched with much interest by all the family and most of the servants; at first the cat would not come to, but we put her in a hamper with plenty of fresh air, and when she *did* come to, the language she used was "something awful," but she soon settled down and made a good recovery. My people were very anxious for me to say I could not go back to the hospital at the end of my fortnight's sick leave as the cat was still in splints, but I had to leave her to my assistant.

Then I returned to duty as Night Sister again, and everything went on much as usual—generally rather more work than I could do well, and sometimes rushing nights of accidents and emergencies, when it seemed almost impossible to fit in all that had to be done.

It seems that every year more operations are done; the cases are sent out more quickly, and so make room for more acute cases, and so the work grows, but the number of nurses does not grow in the same proportion.

In February there was an urgent call for nurses to volunteer for plague duty in India, so I sent in my name—thought it would be a useful experience—and I wasted much time hanging about the India Office for interviews, &c., but eventually they were unkind enough to say I was not strong enough, and refused to send me. *Who* would look very strong after acting for a year as single-handed Night Sister for a hospital of six hundred beds?

Then the authorities made a change, and they decided to increase the night staff by the addition of eight more nurses and one more sister. I was only on for a short time after this came into force, just to set things going, and then I was appointed day sister of M. Ward, the women's surgical ward, where I had worked as a lady pupil, and knew and liked the surgeons so much.

Since I was lady pupil there, and before I was appointed Sister of the ward, they had had several changes of sisters, and no one who had been there long enough to take much interest in it; so there was room for improvement, and the surgeons have been so awfully kind to me that I have had a very nice time.

In that ward my bedroom opened out of my sitting-room (attached to my ward), and we had one very exciting night there.

Since the night staff were increased the nurses have had one meal during the night down in the dining-hall, and there are some probationers who relieve our staff nurses while they go down to this meal. I was fast asleep one night when a probationer rushed into my room, "Oh, Sister, come quick, it's all blazing!" I seized my dressing-gown, and was in the ward in a few seconds thinking that she had set the place on fire with the airing sheets (of course my proper nurse was down at her meal); but it was a house just across a narrow road that was indeed all blazing, and my ward was brilliantly lit up by the flames, and the poor patients were all awake, and some of them quite terrified.

I turned on all the lights, so that they should not see the glare, and then we did our best to reassure them that there was no danger. Two poor women with fractured femurs and their legs slung up to Hodgin splints had already hopped out of their beds, and were literally tied by the leg, and they were all begging for their clothes; so I let two convalescents go to the clothes cupboard and put round the clothes to each bed, or dressing-gowns for the helpless ones, while we got our fire-hose out in case of need; but the firemen very soon got the fire under.

Two of our students, who lived in the house which was on fire, had to jump for their lives, and lost all their belongings, and one of them broke his leg.

It was really a bit alarming, as the ward got so hot and smoky, but the patients soon settled down again, and after we had readjusted splints, &c., no one was any the worse.

I had to take my month's holiday in June this year, rather earlier than I like (as it always seems more difficult to work when you come back to face all the hot weather), but we can't all have our holidays in the best months.

A young brother and a sister and I agreed to spend a fortnight about our old haunts in Switzerland, and we had such a jolly time together.

Of course we went first to Paris, and were fascinated with the shops, but tore ourselves away from them to visit the venerable Notre Dame, and then to spend a little time in the Louvre, but it was only time enough just to make us determined to stay longer in Paris on our way back. In the afternoon we took one of the boats up the Seine, and afterwards went for a walk in the Bois de Boulogne—a delightful breathing-place for the Parisiennes—good roads, lovely trees, and greenery, and yet quite near to all the bustle of the town.

The next day we had a hot and dusty journey on to Geneva, rather afflicted by the presence of some old ladies who wished to keep all the windows shut —it is strange how these petty discomforts fix themselves in one's mind!

At Geneva we had vast, big rooms just looking over the lake, in the Hotel des Bergues, and we took a Sabbath-day's rest there, finding a nice service in the English church, and for the rest of the day wandering about near the lake and up the river.

The next day we felt more energetic, and B. went off for a trip round the lake by steamer, while we went up Salève by steam and electric tram, a lazy way of proceeding, but it was rather an exciting journey crawling up the face of the mountain, and then such a view from the top; mountains, mountains everywhere, and grand old Mont Blanc poking his head over the top, and down below the lake so still and blue, with green trees down to its edge, and then the trees growing darker as they grow higher up, until they stop and the snow-line begins.

The next day we moved on to Chamonix; the train went only as far as Cluses, and from there we had a drive of twenty-five miles by diligence.

It was a delightful drive on a bright, sunny day; at every turn we seemed to get fresh views of Mont Blanc, and each view seemed more beautiful than the last.

We walked a good part of the way while the horses climbed the hills, and we found many varieties of wild flowers and plenty of wild strawberries.

Chamonix is a charming place, but one wanted more time just to loaf about and enjoy the views. The Mer de Glace is, perhaps, the most noted glacier in Switzerland; it is within easy distance of Chamonix (about two hours' walk), and it is a wonderful sight, but somehow I can't describe it, it is all too solemn and grand. I always feel the truth of what the Psalmist says about the men that go down to the sea in ships: "These men see the works of the Lord and His wonders in the deep," and I think the same applies to those who climb into the heights of the mountains, but I suppose he had not had that opportunity!

We left Chamonix with regret, and walked from there over the Col de Balme to Martigny; I think it was about twenty miles, but you can walk twice as far in Switzerland as you can in England without being tired, the air is so clear and bracing. It was a lovely tramp, beautiful flowers and ferns, and rushing streams and waterfalls; the last part of the way was trying, as it was very steep going down into Martigny, and the path was paved with little cobbles, so that we arrived rather footsore.

From there we trained to Glion, a very favourite place with us, just perched above Chillon, with lovely views of Lake Leman, of Chillon Castle, and the fine old Dent de Midi at the end of the lake, and it is within easy walking distance of Montreux. There are many nice walks and climbs about Glion, and the flowers—gentians, narcissi, &c.—were perfectly lovely.

Then we had to turn homewards, and found that we could spare only one night again in Paris (we had meant to stay longer): still it gave us a little more time to examine the treasures of the Louvre.

We had a small excitement in the afternoon. We had been walking through the flower market when a shower of rain came on. We sheltered under one of the stalls, and while we were there we heard what we thought was a sharp clap of thunder, but it proved to be a bomb exploding in the Place de la Concorde, but no one was seriously hurt.

When we got back to London it was very busy with preparations for the Queen's Diamond Jubilee, which was duly celebrated with much rejoicing all over the country before I returned to work in town.

Now, I had better explain why I am leaving here. I have promised to go as nurse to one of the hotels up the Nile (either to Luxor or Assouan, where they always have a doctor and one nurse through the winter season), with a patient who has spent the last eight winters in Egypt. He is now very ill, and still he wants to go, as he can live so much more comfortably in that climate. His mother can't go with him at present, and they can't bear to let him go alone, so I have promised to go to see him through the voyage (we are going by long sea) and to be at hand in case he should get worse before his mother can join him.

You know I love travelling, so in a way I am glad, but I don't think I am fitted for private nursing, and I am a bit nervous, and also it will be anxious work if my patient gets worse out there, but somehow I could not refuse. It is just horrid saying good-bye to every one and everything here.

I will write again soon from the sunny south.

XIX

Here we are in lovely sunshine (the thermometer at 80° in the shade), just on the edge of the desert, and quite contented to rest a while (after a very anxious voyage) before we move on up the Nile.

We sailed from London on October 1st, and had a smooth trip down the Channel, but I soon found my patient was much more of an invalid than I had expected, and was afraid he would get cold before we got into a warmer climate.

The first Sunday out we ran into a dense fog off Cape Finisterre, and our morning service was somewhat disturbed by the constant hooting of the foghorn; some of the passengers jumped up from their knees at each hoot, and the captain cut the service rather short and went up on the bridge. In a couple of hours we emerged into lovely sunshine, which soon dried the wet decks and awnings, but the next day, as we were putting on full steam to get into Gibraltar before sunset, we again ran into a thick bank of fog, and eventually had to change our course and put out to sea until the morning, as they are not allowed to run through the Straits after sunset.

The next morning I was up on deck before five, just as we were running into Gibraltar, and to watch the sun rise from behind the great rock was a most impressive sight.

We had a pleasant trip down the Mediterranean until we entered the Gulf of Lyons, and then the wind got up, and there was a nasty cross sea which made most of us feel squeamish and not sorry when we anchored at Marseilles early one morning; but there we had to tranship to a smaller steamer, and it was raining and cold, and when we got on board the *Clyde* we found they were still coaling, and that the lighter with all our baggage on board was not likely to come for some time, so we could not establish ourselves in our cabins. As there seemed no comfortable place on the boat, we concluded the best thing to do was to take a cab and drive up to a hotel to get warm. Then I went out to buy fresh cream and grapes, and to find out exactly at what time it was necessary to be on board.

I shall never forget the storm of that night after we left Marseilles. I tried to make some hot arrowroot; with much patience I managed it over a spirit lamp, which I wedged into my washing basin with supports; of course the tin of milk could not be trusted to sit on the top of the lamp, so I had to hold it there, and it was not an easy matter as I was flung from side to side in my cabin; then I found that a linseed poultice was indicated, so I again retired to my cabin and wrestled with the spirit lamp, and thought how little one appreciates the conveniences of a modern hospital until one has to do without them.

After that the groans and fearsome noises from other cabins around us were very bad, and I, who have always prided myself on being a good sailor, actually succumbed for an hour or two; but I dragged myself up again in the early hours of the morning to make another poultice, and by breakfast-time the sea began to go down, and the sun came out, but it was several days before some of the passengers crawled up on deck, looking like limp rags, and the tables in the saloon were very empty until just before we reached Alexandria.

We stayed some hours at Malta, and I had an interesting drive round the place.

From Alexandria we had meant to go straight on to Cairo, but eventually agreed it was best to stay a night at a hotel in Alexandria to rest before the dusty train journey.

We had a wretched night, and, not knowing how to find a good doctor if I needed one, I felt very lonely in a vast hotel where no one seemed to speak English.

The next day we managed to journey on to Cairo in the morning, and rested at Shepherd's Hotel until the evening, and then moved on to this place— about half an hour by rail from Cairo, and actually on the borders of the desert.

We have many friends in Cairo, and there is a good train service, so they often come out to spend the day with us, or for the afternoon, and then sometimes I go into Cairo to do necessary shopping or to pay some visits. Cairo is a very gay place, and the people very pleasant and friendly.

One day I went to lunch with some friends, and they drove me to see the Citadel (driving all through the native quarter of the town), and then we had tea with the sisters at the Military Hospital—a rambling big place, designed for a palace and not for a hospital—and they seemed very full up with enteric patients.

Then we went to see the Mosque, and were seized by the feet by several Arabs, who tied on sandals for us before we went inside, and in these we were allowed to flop about. The Mosque is a vast dome, nearly all marble and alabaster, with a lovely alabaster fountain, where the people wash their feet before going in to pray.

We walked all round the fortifications, and had a splendid view of Cairo, and then drove back to town just in time to see the Khedive arrive from Alexandria; a stout, sad-looking young man, his native escort very smart, and riding such beautiful little horses.

Another day I was invited to bicycle out from Cairo to Mena House; so I went into Cairo by the early morning train, and mounted a hired bicycle for the nine-mile ride to Mena House Hotel. The first two miles seemed very perilous, as our route lay all through the town, and many water-carts made the roads very slippery, and electric trams and steam trams rushed about in a most confusing way, and natives in swarms (many of them blind) seemed to take a pleasure in strolling in our track, and stupid donkeys and sad-eyed camels with unwieldy loads kept turning about in unexpected directions, and looking at us in a reproachful way, as much as to say they thought bicycles *quite* out of place in their country.

The narrow bridges over the Nile were thick with traffic, and I was quite glad when we got out to the open country and on to a good road with trees all along.

We left our bicycles at the hotel, and walked out to the great Ghizeh Pyramids, really a most marvellous sight.

The big Pyramid covers as much ground as Lincoln's Inn Fields; enormous blocks of stone, apparently just tumbled one on the top of the other, and yet the whole worked into such perfect shape. To think of how they can have brought these vast blocks of stone down, without mechanical help, from Upper Egypt (for there was no such stone to be found near there) is indeed wonderful.

The Temple, also, is a thing to marvel at, great blocks of granite and alabaster cut and fitted together so perfectly, the doorway as straight as possible, and to think that all this work was done from 3000 to 5000 years ago and is still as sound as ever.

We had not time to climb the Pyramid, but of course we paid our respects to the Sphinx, and wished we could stay to see her by moonlight, when she is said to be even more impressive than in the daylight.

They gave us a very good lunch on the balcony of the hotel, which is said to be the best managed in Egypt; and I should think it would be a very pleasant place to stay at, nice airy rooms and a lovely marble swimming-bath at the back.

As we rode back there was a good deal of wind against us, and I was out of practice and rather tired, so I found the crowded streets of Cairo alarming, and was much relieved to give up my bicycle without having run over any one or damaged the machine.

I think there was more of a crowd than usual, as the Khedive had driven to the station to meet the King of Siam, and we saw the whole procession pass on their way back to the palace.

The King of Siam was very gorgeous in a white uniform with much gold lace, and his two sons were a somewhat curious contrast to the natives around, in their Eton suits and top-hats; they are going up the Nile on a private boat.

Helouan is beginning to fill up for the season (we were about the first arrivals), and we have many visitors. We are in comfortable lodgings, quite on the outskirts of the village; the servant who chiefly waits upon us is a fine Arab with a black moustache, who stalks about in a white night-gown down to his heels, tied round with a red sash; he wears a red fez cap with a blue tassel, and red sandals on his feet; he does most of the housework, for which purpose he puts a housemaid's apron with a bib over his night-gown! His name is "Abdul" (the "slave of God"); and there is a small Arab boy called "Ishmael," who runs messages, and is most interested in our doings.

The mosquitoes are pretty bad at night here, and we have to sleep in nets. Last week we had two days with a south wind blowing, and then the beasts —creeping, crawling, and flying—*were* a trial; there were great wasps (quite three times as large as English ones), and horrid little beasts that look like bugs (only they fly and don't bite) settling on our dinner-table;—I am sure the south wind must have been blowing in the time of the plagues of Egypt!

I am busy collecting things that we want to take up the Nile for our house, as we shall then be 450 miles from the nearest shop, and it is rather difficult, as I don't know at all what the house is like.

There are so many things that I should like to do and see in Cairo, but I have not time, as we are leaving by the first tourist steamer that goes up the Nile, and I don't like to be out for any length of time, but I did manage a visit to the great native hospital, the Kasr-el-Aini, where I know several of the sisters.

It is a very fine place with a very up-to-date theatre; the nurses are all natives (men for the male patients), but they all work under the English sisters.

The sisters have a most delightful Home, their dining and drawing rooms are very spacious apartments, and they each have a very large room, which most of them screen off into bed and sitting rooms.

There is a special fund which provides a carriage and pair for their use, and they have a very good tennis court in their garden, in which they are "At Home" one day each week, and the Cairo people go to tea with them and to play tennis.

I have not told you a word about the native bazaars and all the quaint sights of the Cairo streets, but every one writes about them, and I find them too dazzling to describe. I could sit for hours on the balcony at Shepherd's Hotel just doing nothing but watch the people. Take my advice, and come to see Cairo some day, for it is a most fascinating place, and I am quite loth to leave it.

XX

LUXOR, UPPER EGYPT,
December 1897.

Once more we have moved our camp, and though we managed the move with very little exertion for my patient, and are now settled in very comfortable quarters here, and he is pleased to be amongst old friends and in his old haunts, and the climate is perfectly beautiful, still it is sad to see that he is going downhill; so it has been arranged for his mother and younger brother to join us here, and we are counting the days till they arrive.

We came up the Nile on *Rameses III.*, the newest of Cook's tourist steamers, a very comfortable boat with nice airy cabins. I took all our baggage on board in Cairo, but we had agreed it was better to avoid the noise and bustle of embarking in Cairo, and that we should join the boat when she anchored a few miles away from Helouan, at a place called Badrachin.

Two of our doctor friends had meant to come to see us safely on board, but at the last moment they were both prevented, so we started off in an arabeyeh, escorted by a policeman mounted on a donkey, who had been sent to give us any help he could.

Much to my anxiety, before we had gone far, the sun had disappeared, and a sand-storm had got up, and by the time we had reached the Nile it was quite cold, and the water was very rough with white waves showing.

Rameses III. was anchored at Sakkarah on the other side of the river, but our policeman rode on and signalled to them, and as soon as they saw us they sent off a boat to take us across; it was rather a perilous trip as the boat was a light one, and we shipped a good deal of water. I was thankful when we got safely on board, and found a good doctor and other friends to help us.

The tourists—of whom there were not many, as this was the first trip of the season—were all away sightseeing at the Sakkarah Pyramids.

Strolling up the river on these steamers is a very pleasant way of travelling. Though the banks of the Nile are flat and there is a certain sameness about them, the lights are so wonderful that they never *look* the same. I used to think that the only thing that it was really worth while having to get up early for was a day's hunting, but now I must add the sight of the sunrise on the Nile, and as for the sunsets they are simply gorgeous, the intense red, gold, and orange as the sun sinks with the delicate blue above; and then you turn your back on the sun and face the rich indigo blue of the afterglow, and then in a few minutes it is all dark (no twilight here), and there is a solemn hush over everything.

The steamers don't travel at night, and they stop at various points where there are interesting things to be seen, and then all the tourists troop off and mount the excellent donkeys, who seem to think nothing of the heaviest weights, but canter off to the Tombs or the Temples as though they quite enjoyed it.

I had a very good ride on a big donkey called Mahomet to the Tombs of Beni Hassan, and another day I went ashore and had a good look round Assiout.

On the morning of November 23 I had a long ride out to see the Temple of Dinderah (a very beautiful temple), and then the same evening we reached Luxor just at sunset, and walked up an avenue of palm-trees to the hotel, which just at this season is very empty, so we have large rooms on the ground floor, and there is a delightful garden, where at present we spend most of the day. We have a little house just across the road facing the hotel, and I am very busy getting it ready. As I am the only nurse here, if any visitors should come up ill, I should have to look after them; but so far people are behaving nicely.

We have secured two good Arab boys as servants—Hassan and Girgus. Hassan can speak a little English, but Girgus cannot, and it takes a long time to get much work out of people when you can't talk to them! You would be amused to see me wrestling with Arab carpenters, who seem quite incapable of putting anything up straight, and with Arab painters, who never get the same colour for two days together.

The chaplain's wife, who came up the river with us, has gone on to Assouan for a few days, and as she has left me her donkey to use, I get a little exercise every afternoon.

The other day I had rather an amusing time. I had ridden out to Karnak with Miss L. to see the temple: it was very dusty, and we were very hot; and when we got into the shade of the temple we saw a party of people having tea, with two men in very gorgeous uniforms waiting upon them and a dignified dragoman standing by. I recognised the dragoman as one of Cook's men who had helped us in Cairo, and he gave me a sweeping bow as we passed. I said to Miss L. as we moved away, "I am sure that nice dragoman would like to offer us some tea, and I do want some very badly," and we had not gone very far when the dragoman came after us with a visiting card and "Sir G. N.'s compliments, and would the ladies accept a cup of tea?" so we joined the party and had a most pleasant tea, the dragoman having evidently explained who we were.

They had come up on a dahabeah, and were staying only for one night now, but may return later on. They told us they thought they *must* ride camels in Egypt, so at Keneh they all started off on camels, each with a boy attendant on a donkey, but all except one of the party returned on the donkeys, with the boys on the camels!

The Karnak Temple is very beautiful; I have been to see it several times now, and find something new to gaze at every time I go; once I visited it by moonlight, and then it was most solemn.

There is a very nice little hospital for natives in Luxor, where they do a good many eye and other operations. The native doctor in charge has been most kind in lending me his horse, a perfect little Arab that goes like the wind, and I have had some delightful gallops on the desert.

All the houses in Luxor are built of mud, or mud bricks, the bigger ones being colour-washed over, but often you see a little bit of straw sticking through the colour-wash just to remind you that it is "a house of straw."

We are building a little summer-house out at Karnak, and sometimes drive out there with our lunch and spend the day—the air is fresher away from the village and the cultivated land; and one of the engineers who is building the railway from Cairo to Assouan sometimes lends us his trolley on the line, and a couple of Arabs shove us (with Hassan in attendance) several miles out into the desert. We also do some sailing on the Nile when there is any wind.

Rameses III. stayed here a few days on her way down the river, and most of the passengers came to look us up. One evening they had a fancy dress ball on board. I went down for a little while, and it was such a pretty sight; the boat was moored close in, so that they could dance on deck and then stroll in the hotel grounds, and it was all lit up with Japanese lanterns, and looked so pretty with the palms waving above.

There was a gymkhana one day, and it was very good fun; camel races and buffalo races and all varieties of donkey races; one very amusing race was for gentlemen riding one donkey and driving another with long reins in front of him. The leaders would seldom go straight, and they got hopelessly mixed up in the reins, and had to be disentangled several times.

A favourite amusement here is to play hare and hounds on donkeys. They have quite a big meet of hounds near the hotel, and the hares (three of them) have a long start to give them time to ride out to Karnak, and then they have to try to ride back to the racecourse without being caught.

The hounds are divided into three packs—the fast, the medium, and the slow; the master has to be a man of tact: he sends off with the fast pack the keen young tourists, many of them Americans, the men riding in their shirt sleeves, and they gallop out to the boundary to drive the hares in; then the medium pack trot out in a business-like way, ladies and gentlemen, who are probably very correct in their costume for riding in the Row, and who would not think of riding at home without a top-hat; and, lastly, the slow pack, consisting of people who (in some cases) hardly know a horse from a donkey, and who solemnly jog down to the racecourse and then loiter about to see the fun when the hares come in.

The natives take a great interest in this sport, and call it "hunting the Mahdi," but their sympathies seem to be entirely with the hares, and they give them every assistance by scouting about for the hounds, and secreting the hares and their donkeys in their mud houses when there is danger about.

Dr. R. and I were the hares one day, and we had a most exciting ride, but were caught at last just as we reached the racecourse. At one point I was hustled into a native house (just mud walls with no proper roof), and found a buffalo being milked in one corner and a baby lying on the ground in another, and from there I watched half-a-dozen hounds gallop past, thinking they were close on my heels, and when they got out of sight I doubled off in another direction.

The donkeys seem quite to enter into the fun of the thing, and do their best, but sometimes they get excited and bray—inexcusable behaviour, which is most disconcerting when you are trying to hide in a patch of sugar-cane!

XXI

LUXOR, UPPER EGYPT,
January 1898.

It was difficult for us to realise the snow and cold that you had for Christmas, while we were enjoying perpetual sunshine here.

My patient is now established in his little mud house, just across the road from this hotel. I am thankful to say his mother and brother have arrived, so we share the nursing between us.

It has been downhill work lately, and now he seldom leaves his bedroom, a large "upper chamber" with a nice view over the palm-trees to the Nile.

The nurse from Assouan has come down to be with him at night, as I have been annexed by a poor lady in the hotel who is desperately ill; she came up from Cairo with a very bad throat, and now that is better, but she is still very ill, and it is not quite clear whether it is typhoid fever or general pyæmia, but I am afraid, whatever it is, her strength cannot hold out much longer.

I am with her for all the nights and part of the days, and go backwards and forwards to the house, and get some sleep in just when I can.

There has been much excitement here about the rumour of war in the Soudan, and now it is more than rumour, and the troops are being pushed up country as fast as they can.

Cook's people are in great trouble, as all their tourists going down to Cairo have had to be turned off the boats at Naghamadi (the present railroad head), and they have to go the rest of the way down by train, while the boats turn back to take the troops up to Assouan. Some regiments are being sent all the way by rail, in spite of the line not being yet finished.

The engineers are working day and night. I met one of them just now, who said he was up to his eyes in work, and that he had twenty telegrams in his pocket, all different orders, and each contradicting the one before; so I said I supposed he did what he thought was right and hoped for the best!

They have been busy here with an old tub of a steamer that has been used for years as a landing stage; with much tinkering at last they got the engines to work, and now she has gone wobbling down the Nile to bring up stores. It was exciting when they first lit up the fires, as I hear she ran away and knocked pieces out of the road on the front.

The Oxfordshire and Lincolnshire Regiments have gone past, the men packed like sardines in the boats.

I badly want to go up with them, but at present they don't seem to be sending any sisters, and my work is cut out for me here just at present.

All the steamers that come up, besides being heavily loaded, are towing large barges with either men or stores in them, so there is a good deal of delay about our mails, &c.

I expect you hear more of what is going on at the front than we do, as all the wires are blocked with service messages, and we hear only rumours; to-day we hear our troops have had a bad smash up near Berber, and that they have lost a gunboat, but whether there is any truth in it or not is very doubtful.

To-day the Camerons are passing through here, and the natives are much excited at the kilts. I think they rather imagine that England has run out of men and has begun to send the women!

Somehow life seems very strange here just now; for one thing, there is the rustle and bustle of war in the air, then, at the same time, in this little place we are already having a stern fight against the enemy of disease, and all the time there are tourists filling up the hotel and making merry, and you hear them talk of the Luxor Meet of the Sporting Club, and which donkey they will secure as their mount, as though it was the most important thing in the world.

Until last week I still went for a ride now and then by way of refreshment. There is a doctor here who rides an enormous white Syrian horse, and he was most kind in bringing me a beautiful little Arab, and taking me out for a gallop when I could get away; the Arab was too quick for the Syrian, and often, having let it go, I had to wait for him afterwards. One day we were coming in from the desert and passed our chaplain, who afterwards amused my friends by telling them that I had passed him at such a pace on the Arab that the wind I made nearly blew him off his donkey, and then about a mile behind something thundered past that at first he thought was a white elephant but afterwards concluded it was a watering-pot of a new fashion, as it left such a track of damp on the sand!

One day the German Consul took me to see his collection of curios (I believe he does a good deal of trading in them): he has got a splendid collection. I had to drink native coffee—which I can't abide—but before I left he gave me a beautiful little "antique," a little blue image that was found in a tomb near here, and probably dates from about 3000 B.C., so I forgave him the coffee!

The other day Miss C., the housekeeper at the hotel, knocked up with dysentery, and was very seedy for a few days. Before she got well again there was an urgent call for more steamers for troops; so the steamer *Rameses the Great*, that happened to be moored here (meaning to stay four days while the passengers explored the place), suddenly had to turn all her passengers and their baggage off into the hotels and leave them there, while she did a trip up to Assouan and back. The hotel was simply packed for five days, and the noise was very bad for our sick ones; poor Miss C. was frantic at not being able to get about and see about rooms, &c., for all these people, so I had to do what I could to help her, but I was frightfully busy with so many ill.

The Nile is getting very low and "smelly," and we hear that they have several cases of dysentery at Assouan, and there is a poor lady somewhere up the river on a dahabeah very ill with it, and there is no nurse within reach free to go to her.

With all this urgent traffic on the river it is difficult to get things up from Cairo (even urgent "medical comforts"), and you cannot imagine how many things one finds lacking for the sick ones from day to day, when you are 450 miles from the nearest chemist's shop, with uncertain communication by post or telegraph.

I am always making raids on the little hospital, and the doctor there is most kind in helping us, but he is short of some things that he needs himself and cannot get—for one thing, the supply of chloroform is very nearly exhausted. We sent an urgent message (telegraph not available) by the last boat going up to Assouan, and we hope the doctor there may be able to lend us some for the present.

It seems weeks since I have had a night in bed; my poor lady is so ill that I can hardly leave her, and I just sleep in an arm-chair in her room when her husband sits by her for a time.

The Arab servants, especially Hassan and Girgus, are wonderfully attentive and good—in fact, all help us as much as they possibly can; but with people so desperately ill one does long for London, and the best physicians, and the best nurses to help one. It is not possible to do all one would wish for several patients at once both night and day; and having had so little sleep of late I am afraid of forgetting things, and I have to write all the orders down and tick them off as I carry them out.

This letter has been written in scraps, and I am finishing it as I sit by poor Mrs. ——; I must keep awake somehow till her husband wakes, then he will watch while I have a nap. I fear it is quite hopeless, and she has been unconscious for some hours now, so I cannot leave the poor man alone with her.

XXII

You would gather from my last letter that we were having a sad and trying time at Luxor, and after I posted to you we had so much more of sadness and sorrow that it seems like a bad dream, and I can't write much about it.

The poor lady died of pyæmia, and a few days later my patient was laid to rest in the little cemetery out in the desert that he loved so well.

All the winter the tourists had been so fit and well up the Nile (fortunately for me), but in January every one seemed to get ill, and they had quite an outbreak of dysentery. It began up at Assouan, but two poor young ladies (travelling with a young brother) became very ill between Assouan and Luxor, and were carried ashore and brought to the hotel. Our night nurse went off to nurse them, and as soon as I was free I had to go straight on to help her, as they were both desperately ill.

It was my first experience of tropical dysentery, and in some ways it seemed almost more like cholera—nothing seemed to check it. A very good physician came up from Cairo, and stayed some days trying everything to save them, and nurse and I were working night and day, but it was no use, and they both died within twenty-four hours of each other.

Then others got bad, and we had to go from room to room doing what we could for them, and wishing we either had half-a-dozen nurses, or else had all our patients in one hospital ward. Gradually the others all began to improve, and we were beginning to think of going home, when I was telegraphed for to go up to Assouan to nurse the Bishop of ——, who was very ill; the nurse who was stationed up there also being laid up with dysentery.

I was not pleased at having to go, as we were just packing up to travel home, clearing up the house, &c., and I was feeling very done up, but I could not well refuse, as there was no other nurse within reach; so I went off by the post boat, and spent most of the two days on board in sleeping, as I did not know how much work might be waiting for me, and I had a good deal to make up in the way of sleep. I find from my diary that between the 16th of January and the 3rd of February I had never had a complete night in bed, and sometimes even the odd hours of sleep were very few and far between.

But when I got to Assouan I found that every one was on the mend, and they hardly needed a nurse, so I stayed only a few days to help (and managed to explore Philæ one afternoon), and then I left again by post boat for Cairo, the doctor putting a lady, who had been very ill with dysentery, under my care, and giving me a little stock of medicines to use at my discretion, as the post boats—unlike the tourist boats—carry no doctor.

We stayed an hour or two at Luxor, so that I managed to collect my baggage and said many good-byes. All the inhabitants—including the servant boys and the donkey boys—seemed to be there to see us off, and they had all been so very kind to me through a very trying winter that I felt as though I had known them for years.

There were pleasant people on board the boat, and the gentleman sitting next to me at table knew Kimberley well, and knew my brother out there, so we had much talk about South Africa.

The boat was simply packed; and, as it was getting very hot, every one wanted to rush down the river at the same time. There were supposed to be thirty-two first-class berths, and the manager told me that there were fifty-five passengers on board—men sleeping in all the bathrooms, and the saloon full at night.

I had a sort of little dog-kennel to myself in the second-class—not a bad little hole when I got there, but to get to it each time I had to cross the lower deck, where all the native passengers live and sleep.

My sick lady improved as we got down the river, and it was very lucky she did, as before we reached Cairo I became seedy with dysentery myself, and had to consume some of the drugs the Assouan doctor had given me in case of need.

The last day on board was exciting, as the Nile was so low we kept banging on to sandbanks, and all the glasses were broken; and as many of the passengers had only just allowed time to catch their ship at Alexandria, there was much anxiety lest we should stick fast.

I saw my lady patient safely into good hands at Mena House, and then just caught my friends in Cairo (they had gone down from Luxor when I went up to Assouan), and after getting some advice from one of our good medical friends there, we went straight on to join our ship at Alexandria.

When I got on board I felt so absolutely done up, I had to turn straight into my berth, and the ship's doctor took me in charge. I believe he rather thought I was in for typhoid, and wanted us to go on to Venice with them, so that he could look after me for a bit longer (as they stay some days at Venice), but three days' rest at sea and some medicines pulled me together a bit, and I did not want to upset plans.

We landed at Brindisi, and spent an uncomfortable night in a hotel, because we found the sheets were very wet, and felt obliged to sleep in blankets, a thing I never enjoy.

From there we had a train journey of eleven hours to Naples, and we did an idiotic thing, for which we have not forgiven ourselves yet: we got up at 4.30 A.M., thinking our train started at 6 A.M., and when we got to the station found that our tickets were made out to travel by another route, and the train did not leave till 9.30 A.M.!

Naples was perfectly beautiful; from our windows such a glorious view of the bay and of Vesuvius in the distance. We could not go up Vesuvius as he was rather "active" just then, and some people who went up the day we arrived nearly got burnt with some hot lava.

We went one day by steamer to Sorrento (a place I should like to stay at some day), and then over to Capri, and we explored the wonderful Blue Grotto there. Capri is a sweet place, with such lovely flowers and ferns.

Another day we spent at Pompeii, and wished we could spare more time for exploring the Museum in Naples, where most of the best things from Pompeii are now shown; and then a drive we took along the bay to Posilipo is one of the most beautiful drives I have ever enjoyed.

From Naples we moved on to Rome. It is quite hopeless to try to "see" Rome in anything under a month at least, so we did not try. The place seemed to be full of our Egyptian friends, and we met them at every turn, so we had a very pleasant time there, and of course we did see *some* of the sights.

We spent some time at St. Peter's and several more of the wonderful churches, and we explored the Colosseum, and the Forum, and the Thermæ Caracalla, and we went down some Catacombs (and were very glad to get safely up again!); in fact, we saw just enough to make us wish to return some day with time (and money) to enjoy it all more fully.

We then moved on to Florence and had a few most enjoyable days there; the picture galleries were most fascinating—so many pictures that one has known and loved all one's life (from photographs), and will now love all the more for having seen the originals. The town is very interesting, and the surrounding country is lovely.

Our last day in Florence was wet. This was disappointing, but as it was the first rain I had seen since last September I could hardly complain.

We spent a night in the train, and then stayed a few hours in Milan, just to see the very beautiful cathedral, and then got on board a corridor train to cross the St. Gothard. Near Milan the fields were thick with primroses and anemones, and it was quite hot, but we soon got up amongst the snow, and then the scenery was simply grand.

We stayed a few days with some Swiss friends in Zürich. They have a delightful house looking over the lake, and the snow mountains in the distance are such a restful sight.

One day we went out by train, and then did a little climbing, and got up amongst the snow: it was so funny after all the scorching we have had just lately.

From there we travelled by night on to Paris; and now we have come to the end of our "saunter" across the Continent, and I am sure it has done us all good, and has been most refreshing.

I have just been out to get my hair shampooed, and I think I have now got rid of the last remains of Egyptian dust. To-morrow we make tracks for England, and then I don't quite know what is to be my next move, but more work, I hope, of some kind or another.

XXIII

I don't think I have written to you since I slipped back into my work here.

We got back from Egypt in April, and I spent a little time at home and paid a few visits, and then the Matron asked me if I would return to take charge of one of the women's surgical wards for four months while the sister was away on sick leave; so back I came at the beginning of July, and it seems as though I am likely to remain. I had such a nice welcome back from every one (from the surgeons down to the porters), that I soon felt quite at home again.

At first it was rather strange, as they have changed the "off duty" times, and all the nurses get more time off, so that means you have more nurses, and when they were all on together it seemed such a crowd to me: in that ward for twenty-two beds and four cots I had a staff nurse, a senior probationer, and three other probationers, and two lady pupils, seven besides myself on day duty and a staff nurse and a probationer on night duty; but it is seldom they are all on at the same time, and I have to run around and see that those who are on attend to the work of those who are off, and that things are not neglected because "it is not my work"!

It is nice for the nurses not to be so rushed as we used to be, but I am not quite sure that it is such good training; I don't think they feel quite so personally responsible for their patients' welfare as they did when there was no one equally responsible with them; it is rather difficult to explain exactly what I mean—for one thing, the staff nurses now have two days off together each month, so we have a senior probationer who takes over their work for those two days, and I find they get much more out of touch with what has been ordered for the patients than they did when they were away only for one day; but I am getting used to it now.

The ward I had when I first came back was rather dingy, and I regretted all the nice flower-pots and vases I had left behind in the ward I had when I was last here, to say nothing of my nice stock of children's clothes (I had heaps of white sailor blouse tops for the small boys, and muslin pinafores for the little girls, with pale blue frocks to wear under the pinafores on high days and holidays); but I did not spend much on vanities in that ward, as it was not worth while for a short time, and the more fancy things you have the more it costs you in washing, as the hospital won't pay for vanities, though it does make a difference to the look of your ward when visitors go round, and the mothers just love to see their poor little kiddies dressed up "like a real little lady" instead of in flannelette!

I liked both the night and the day staff nurse in that ward, and they were very nice to me (sometimes staff nurses are *not* nice to a sister doing temporary work, as they often think they might have been allowed to do the sister's work themselves).

The ward had been noted for never being without squalling babies, and I was rather amused to hear from another old nurse of mine that these staff nurses had learnt that I was very particular about tidiness, and very anxious that the babies should have no reasonable excuse for squalling; so they were determined to try to please me in those respects. One day I came down from the theatre (after being up for several operations) just at tea-time, and I thought the ward looked rather untidy, but I wanted my tea so badly and the ward-maid had it all ready for me, so, after taking a look at the operation cases, I—rather unwisely—concluded I would drink it before going round to tidy up, and, of course, before I had finished tea the Matron came in, and I had to escort her round, inwardly fuming at some crumbs by a child's cot, and some of the trays brought down from the theatre and not put tidily away; but Matron was very amiable, and when we got to the door she said, "Sister, I never remember seeing the ward so trim and neat after a theatre afternoon, and not a single baby squalling!"—so of course I told the staff nurse, and she was mightily pleased.

We had had a curious case in the theatre that afternoon—a poor little scrap of a baby, one day old, born with an imperforate anus; as soon as they began to give it an anæsthetic it stopped breathing, and after trying to revive it for some time the surgeon put on his coat and went away, but we continued doing artificial respiration, and eventually the child came round; so another surgeon (who was still in the hospital) came in, and he advised the house surgeon to do colostomy, which he did very rapidly, and the poor little mite was relieved, but it only lived a day.

We had a first-rate house surgeon on just then, and he looked after his dressers well. You have no idea how slack and lazy the dressers sometimes get if the house surgeon is not keen, and it makes a vast difference to the patients' comfort.

It happened to be our "take in" week when Bank Holiday came, and we had a very lively week. Altogether we took in sixteen cases, but a few of them were injuries to arms or fingers, so they were able to go out again after a night or two, thus leaving beds free for others.

On Bank Holiday itself things were pretty quiet until the evening, and then we had four accidents in two hours—an old lady of seventy-nine with a fractured femur, a baby with a scalp wound (fell from its chair on to the fender), a little child badly scalded, and a very big and fat woman with a fractured tibia and fibula, who, I was horrified to find, was expecting a baby to arrive very shortly, and as none of my nurses had had any experience of such things, nor had the present night sister, I felt obliged to keep within hail both night and day; but one Sunday I thought it seemed safe to go out to church, and another sister promised to attend if required, and sure enough she *was* required, but all went well, and the mother made a good recovery, and I think was rather pleased to go out with a fine healthy baby, having been saved all the expense of her confinement.

When the sister of that ward returned, there was a small men's accident ward vacant, so I was offered that until a larger ward should be free.

I was sorry to leave the children, but the new ward was under the surgeons for whom I had worked before I went to Egypt, and I was glad to be on for them again.

It was November when I moved my camp, and I seemed to have hardly had time to turn round before Christmas was upon us, and a very bright and cheery Christmas we had, in spite of the fact that we were "taking in," and the cases simply streamed in. Altogether we admitted twenty-one cases during the week for our twenty beds. Of course some kept going out, but we had to send our most movable patients to sleep in other wards, so as to keep a bed always ready for the next accident.

Amongst the cases we had two poor fellows who had cut their throats; one a lad of twenty-one who had had influenza, and the other a man of thirty-two who had been jilted by a girl. They both had tracheotomy done, and both did pretty well at first, but I don't think the younger man wanted to get better, and eventually he got pneumonia and died. The other man got all right again. All through Christmas week they both had policemen sitting by them in case they should attempt suicide again, and these policemen were most useful in helping with the decorations.

At the same time we had a big drayman in, who had fallen off his dray and got slight concussion of the brain. He did not get quite sensible for some time (though he was never very ill), and he was always trying to get out of bed, and whenever any one got up on the ladders to do a little decorating there would be a call that "No. 10 was getting out," and we all had to run to put him back and tuck him up again.

These various interruptions made our decorations a very slow process, but eventually the ward looked very nice, and I think the patients had a very happy Christmas; even the two poor cut-throat men seemed quite pleased and interested in their presents, though they were neither of them able to enjoy the privilege of a smoke, which all the other men (including the policemen) so much enjoyed on Christmas Day.

One man who came in with a damaged knee told me that he was a rival "strong man" to Sandow; and, as he was verging on delirium tremens for some days, we felt a little anxious until he calmed down; but he proved to be quite a nice patient.

XXIV

I seem to have been wasting a lot of time this year in being seedy in one way or another, so I don't think that I have much of interest to write to you about, and now that the war in South Africa is making us all excited (as every one feels as if he ought to lend a hand), it is difficult to think of the trifles that have been filling up our lives for the last few months.

After I wrote to you last, we had in yet another cut-throat who proved to be a lunatic, and he gave us a very lively time before we got him well enough to despatch to an asylum. One day he jumped out of bed in a great hurry (as he was very fond of doing if the policeman in charge took his eye off him for a minute), so the man in the next bed called out "Halloa, mate, where are you off to?" to which he replied, "I've got a second-class pass for heaven, so I'm off," and it took some persuasion before he would believe that the train for that destination was not due yet. Another night he proposed to the night nurse, as he thought they might get on well in "the fried fish line" together! It is strange how nervous men are with any one a little bit "off": even some of these big policemen always call out for us to come if a man gets restless. I am not a bit afraid of them, and can generally get them to do what I want with a little chaff; but I am heartily tired of having cut-throats in the ward: I seem to have had so many of them at one time or another, and they are a great anxiety.

We had so many accidents in from the railway station near by last winter that the Superintendent very kindly told me (as one of the accident sisters) I might have a free pass any week-end that I liked to apply for it to any station on their line; so I had a very good time going to visit friends and relations at the seaside when I was able to get away from Saturday to Monday; and they were first-class passes too, so that one could go by the fastest trains.

One evening in May I found that a lad, who had been brought in with a broken leg, was peeling nicely all over, and we extracted a history that *might* have meant a slight attack of scarlet fever, but it was so indefinite that the house surgeon did not believe it, and did not have him moved at once; and two days later another small boy developed scarlet fever, and then one of the nurses, and they began to talk about closing the ward; then one day I had a raging headache, but did not think anything of it, but when I went to bed (much to my disgust) I found I had a brilliant rash; and the next day the doctor came along and agreed in my diagnosis of scarlet fever, and offered to isolate me there or send me to the London Fever Hospital (paying), but I thought I would just as soon sample an ordinary M. A. B. Hospital, so I took my departure in state in the fever ambulance, with a crowd of friends to see me off—from a safe distance—at the door.

They made me very comfortable at the Fever Hospital, but I felt rather a fraud, as I had the fever so very mildly that I was never ill at all: no sore throat and no temperature after the first two days—in fact I think they doubted whether I had ever had it at all, and it was very slow work waiting to peel. Having at last accomplished this process, I went back to the Hospital to clear up my rooms, as a larger ward was going to be vacant soon, and Matron wanted me to have it after I had taken a holiday.

So I had a good time at home in the best of the summer weather, and paid a few visits, going down to the Isle of Wight and having some splendid bathing and boating there; but it is strange how it takes it out of one having scarlet fever, even when you have it as ridiculously mildly as I did, and I had a good deal of trouble with swollen feet and other forms of feebleness.

In July I attended a very pleasant function at Marlborough House, when the Princess of Wales presented me with my certificate of membership of the Royal National Pension Fund for Nurses, and I met many old friends amongst the one thousand odd nurses who were there.

It was a scorching hot day, and there were some active non-commissioned officers of the Scots Guards who had their work cut out in marshalling the crowd of nurses for their march past; and we found it warm work standing in the sun, as we were wearing indoor uniform, and our caps were not much protection; but as soon as that was over we found plenty of shade under the beautiful trees, and were provided with ices and delicious plates of fruit and other refreshments.

I knew a member of the household, and she very kindly took me round some of the royal apartments, and it was interesting to peep into the cool dining-room, with the lunch ready laid for the royalties to partake of as soon as they had dismissed us, but they stayed chatting with some of the nurses for some time, and altogether we spent a very pleasant time there.

As I was travelling home afterwards in an express train we were suddenly pulled up with a tremendous jerk that threw us and our baggage about the carriage, and when we had picked ourselves up and could look out of the window, we discovered that our carriage was on fire. Fortunately a signalman had noticed it, and telegraphed to the next signal-box to stop the train; we all had to bundle out at a country siding, and the carriage was taken off to be attended to by the men there, while we and our baggage were packed into the rest of the train—which already seemed quite full— and then we hurried on again; but if the signalman had not noticed it, it might have been very unpleasant for us.

I went back to work early in August, and when I got to the Hospital the doctor who generally looks after me was away. It never struck me that I needed to see a doctor, and the Matron did not think to suggest it, so I took over my new ward and began to get things into shape and to my liking. It seemed to me that it was very hard work, but I just put it down to the fact that the weather was very hot, and that I had been slacking for so long; and I thought I must pull myself together; but in about a fortnight the doctor returned, and next day he came to see me and said I was not fit for work yet; so, much to my disgust, I was bundled off for more rest.

Towards the end of September I again got into harness, worked for about a fortnight, and then knocked up with acute neuritis in my head, with herpes, &c. I *was* cross, but the pain in my head was too bad for me to worry about anything else. I was warded in a medical ward, given big doses of morphia at pretty frequent intervals, and generally fussed over, as I had the honour of being a "very interesting and unusual case." When my head got better the pain started down my legs—sciatica—so they kept me in bed for some time, and when I got up I was rather a wreck, and they said I must go south;

so once more I went off to stay with some relations near Southampton, and it was the middle of November before I eventually got back to work. Just fancy having to take from May to November to get over scarlet fever and its effects, especially when the fever lasted only about a couple of days. Of course every one who came to see me after I got back, wanted to know how long I had been at work, as they supposed I should be sent off duty for something else before I had worked a fortnight!

While I was down near Southampton, I went once or twice to the docks to see the first troops going off to South Africa. The men looked very fit and trim in their new khaki suits, but they were very tight packed on the troopships and liners. One day I saw the *Kildonan Castle* off with 2400 men on board; crowds of people to see them off, and *such* cheering and singing of "Auld Lang Syne" and "God Save the Queen." Some of them looked such boys to go out and rough it at the front, and it is sad to think that they can't all come back—one wonders how many?

I wish I could go too. Opinions seem divided as to whether the war will soon be over or not.

XXV

R.M.S. "Tantallon Castle,"
March 1900.

I couldn't stand it any longer; all my friends were going off to the front; and, though many people said the war would be over before they landed, we kept hearing accounts of how bad the enteric was, and that the nurses were being overworked, so I felt I must at least offer to lend a hand.

I was afraid if I sent in my papers in the ordinary way I might get sent to a home station to free some Army Sister to go out, and that would not have suited me at all, so I thought I would go down to the War Office, and see for myself if I could get sent to the front.

About the middle of January I boldly went down and asked to see the Secretary of the Army Medical Department. I quite expected to be told I could not do so without an appointment, but I think the orderly must have thought I *had* an appointment, for he showed me into a waiting-room, and there a strange thing happened: there were several people waiting, and amongst them a gentleman whose face I thought I knew, but I could not remember where I had met him before. After a few minutes he came up to me and said, "I think you are Miss L.?" and I said I had been trying to think whether we had met before, and where? and then he reminded me of how we had travelled down the Nile on the same post boat in 1898, and had talked of South Africa then, as he knew of my brother out there. Then he said, "But what do you want here?" and I replied, "Like every one else, I want to get sent out to the Cape." After he had meditated for a few minutes he said, "Well, I'm offering to give them a field hospital of one hundred beds, and to run it for three months at the Cape. If they accept it, will you go with it?" Of course I said I would like a shot; and then he was sent for to see the Secretary, and I waited and waited, and thought he must have forgotten all about me; but at last an orderly came to say, "The Secretary wished to see Miss ———," and the people who had been waiting longer than I had glared at me, as I was escorted to the Secretary's room.

There I found my friend of the Nile still talking to the Secretary, and the Secretary turned to me with a frown, and asked me what I meant by coming down to the War Office without an appointment, instead of sending for the application forms in the usual way? So I told him I did not intend to apply in the usual way, and risk being sent to some home station. I had too good a berth in England to give it up for that, but that if I found they would give me a chance of service at the front I would be glad to go and do what I could; that I knew South Africa, and knew what to expect in the way of climate, and knew how to manage the native servants, and so on.

Then he melted a little, and said, "Well, this gentleman has been most liberal in offering us a complete hospital, which we are going to accept, and he has asked for you to go with it, so if you will send in your papers and testimonials in the usual way you will stand a very good chance of success." Did you ever hear of such a piece of good luck? If I had not gone down personally to the War Office, I should never have met my friend of the Nile, and if I had even gone five minutes later I should never have met him; and afterwards, if I had seen in the papers about his giving a hospital, I should never have thought of applying to go with it, as, when we met on the Nile, I barely knew his name, and should never have connected him with the hospital.

I asked him the other day what made him give me this chance on the spur of the moment, and he told me that he did not wish to leave the appointment of the staff entirely to the Government, and he did not personally know any fully-trained nurse whom he could ask, and he thought if I had a quarter of the brains he knew my eldest brother to possess I should be a good help to him.

I have had heaps of congratulations, as every one says that, though many sisters and nurses have gone from our hospital, this is the best appointment of any that has come our way.

I sat up most of that night filling up papers required by the War Office, and copying out testimonials to send in with them; also writing home, as I had not even told them I was applying to go.

For the next day or two my ward was very heavy with bad cases, and took up most of my time and thoughts; but on the third day I was sent for, and told I was not only accepted but had been appointed Lady Superintendent, and was to select five sisters to go with me, and send their names in for approval. They hoped we should sail in about three weeks.

Then followed a very busy time; the authorities of my hospital were most kind in being willing to let me go, but the fact that so many sisters and nurses were leaving for the front was causing a great scarcity of seniors, so I felt obliged to stay as long as I possibly could, only going home for a long week-end to say good-bye.

There were shoals of letters (sent for me to deal with) of nurses and others wishing to go with us. Some of them were amusing: one was from a viscountess, another from a member of a theatrical troupe; a large proportion of the applicants had had no training, but were "willing to learn"; some offered to pay their own expenses if I would only act as their chaperon—they seemed to think we were going out for a picnic.

However, there were plenty of applications from well and fully-trained nurses, and the chief difficulty was to know which to leave out.

I had to attend at the War Office for an interview with the Selection Committee. Princess Christian was one serving on this committee, and she came and shook hands with me and was most kind.

All the sisters whose names I had sent in were duly appointed to the Army Nursing Service Reserve; and then, having settled the staff, I had to help in choosing the fittings and stores for the hospital, as they wished to take out everything so as to be quite independent when we landed wherever we might be sent.

Lengthy lists had to be made out of bowls and porringers, thermometers, splints, crutches, charts and chart-cases, syringes, bedding and linen, shirts, suits for convalescents, scrubbing and other brushes, tanks for disinfecting linen, &c.

There are so many things that seem to come by nature in England which it would be most trying to find oneself without on the other side.

And then there were the food supplies to be ordered: flour, sugar, all groceries, invalid foods, &c.—in fact everything, and enough of everything, to last for at least three months.

Having chosen all the fittings we could possibly think of, we found great difficulty in getting room on board ship to despatch our cargo, as men were being so urgently called for, and the ships were going out packed with regiments and their baggage.

In the intervals of running a heavy surgical ward, selecting sisters, and choosing stores, I had to get my uniform made and buy a suitable kit for a hot climate; I also bought a second-hand saddle (which I knew would be useful wherever we were stationed), and had it packed in a tin-lined case, which took a good many other things inside the saddle, and I thought if we were living in tents the case would be useful to save some of my goods from the white ants.

The hours I could give to sleep were few in those weeks, but I shall make up arrears on board ship.

We had various false alarms as to the date of sailing, all of which I had to communicate to the sisters and then contradict!

I left the hospital on February 22nd with many regrets, after six years' work, having been a Sister, or a Night Sister, or an Assistant Matron there for the last five years.

We thought we were going to sail at once, but in the end it was decided that the medical officers and the orderlies would have to leave a few days before the sisters. I was sorry for this, as I had hoped to get to know them a little on board ship.

Before they sailed, Mr. X., who was providing the hospital, gave a dinner party to all the staff, and we had a most pleasant evening. After the dinner there was a large reception, and I was introduced to many people whose names are well known both in South Africa and in England.

The doctors sailed on February 28th, and on March 1st I was at the Army and Navy Stores doing a little final shopping when the news came that Ladysmith was relieved; the excitement was intense; such cheering and waving of flags, and they set all the musical boxes, &c., to play "Rule Britannia"!

Mr. X. had decided to go out with us to see the hospital erected, and on March 3rd we sailed from Southampton on the R.M.S. *Tantallon Castle.*

We have troops on board, and I shall never forget the cheering the people at Southampton gave us as we got away.

The first-class is full up with officers and some "gentlemen troopers" of the Yeomanry.

We are now ploughing down the Channel with the sea so calm few people can even think of being sea-sick, so I thought I would send you a yarn up-to-date, and then you would understand that it has been impossible for me to come to say good-bye.

Until we reach Cape Town, we don't know what our destination will be; in the meantime I am having a good rest, and shall be quite fit for any amount of work by the time we land.

I hope to post this at Madeira.

XXVI

That was a strange voyage out on the *Tantallon Castle*. For one thing, instead of the usual mixed lot of passengers, the boat was nearly full of soldiers; there were very few ladies on board besides one Army Superintendent Sister with a batch of sisters and my little party of six, also a few wives of the senior officers; there were practically no old people or children on board.

As one would expect, with so many young men on board (many of them mere boys), there was a great deal of fun and joking, and yet beneath it all there was an under-current of solemnity.

I think we all felt that it was not possible that we should all return (before we left we heard how many were dying of enteric and dysentery), and we hoped, if we were to be left behind, we should have a chance of doing a bit before we got knocked over. Very few of the officers had ever been under fire, and they felt it was going to be a very new experience, and some of them talked of it with awe. I don't mean that they were the least bit "funky," but they wondered whether they would be certain to remember how to manage their men and lead them on as steadily as if they were on parade; some of them thought they would be sure to duck their heads when the bullets were flying, and it would "look so jolly bad."

We played the usual games on board, but in the morning the upper decks were given up to the men, who drilled and did physical exercises to keep them fit. At the request of Colonel H., we sisters held some classes on "first aid." About thirty officers put down their names as wishing to learn, and attended for half an hour every morning, and we taught them simple bandaging, how to stop hæmorrhage, and how to apply improvised splints, &c.

At Madeira we could not get much in the way of news from the front, so we supposed that nothing very exciting had happened yet; we had a few hours ashore to stretch our legs, and paid a visit to the fruit market.

There was an American man-of-war anchored close to us, and when we left she manned her yards, and the men cheered tremendously, and her band played "Rule Britannia."

There were three deaths on board during the voyage, all reservists, and all from pneumonia; it seemed so awfully sad that they should have given up their homes and everything to come out, and then have got knocked over before they had even seen the enemy or fired a shot. I heard that these men were ill before they came on board, but would not report themselves in case they should be left behind, and they came on board straight from their beds in bitter cold.

I have never been to sea in such a crowded ship before; there were four in my cabin, and in a week or two at sea you get to know the good and bad points of your cabin mate's character better than in several months ashore.

At our table there was a Captain —— in charge of a company of "Gentlemen Yeomanry," who were going out, paying all their own expenses: it was rather strange for him having his troopers travelling in the first saloon. He had been in the army, but had given it up because he could not get five months free for hunting, besides some shooting and fishing!

There was another captain also at our table who had been A.D.C. to General Kitchener in the Soudan campaign, and was going out to join him again; he had seen a lot of service, and was very interesting.

Amongst the soldiers in the third-class there are two District Messenger boys going out as trumpeters for the Cape Mounted Rifles.

Most of the officers and some of the soldiers were inoculated against typhoid during the voyage. But for a scarcity of lymph we also should have been inoculated, to avoid waste of time after our landing, but we gave it up, as it was more important for the men who would probably be sent straight up country.

Sunday on board was kept very quietly; it was good to see a large attendance at the Holy Communion service in the early morning, and the parade service was a very hearty one; we had the well-known hymns, "Lead, Kindly Light," and "Onward, Christian Soldiers," and then one that I did not know so well, beginning "O Lord, be with us when we sail," and containing the two following verses, which seemed especially appropriate:

"If duty calls from threaten'd strife
  To guard our native shore,
And shot and shell are answering fast
  The booming cannon's roar,

Be Thou the main-guard of our host,
  Till war and danger cease;
Defend the right, put up the sword,
  And through the world make peace."

The last night on board we had a farewell dinner-party, not sitting at our usual places, but making little parties of our friends. Whenever I go for a voyage, I think there is something a little sad when it comes to an end, and we all part and go our different ways, but there was something especially sad in saying good-bye to all these bright young fellows, who had to go off to "face the shot and shell."

We landed at Cape Town on 20th March, and found that the troopship, with our medical officers on board, had arrived only that morning, though they sailed some days before we did; they had had a good deal of illness on board, and had to send nearly fifty men into hospital at Cape Town, and they had had two deaths during the voyage.

Soon after we got into dock I received orders to take our sisters and their baggage up to a boarding-house in Roeland Street. This we accomplished with the help of the agents, who rejoice in the name of Divine, Gates & Co.; but we had not been established there very long when I received further orders that we should rejoin our ship in a day or two, as our beds were more urgently required round in Natal than in Cape Colony.

Cape Town was in a great state of excitement; martial law was in force, and armed patrols were riding about, and there were constant rumours that the Boers were close to the Cape.

The docks were crowded with men, horses, and stores, all being disembarked, and sent up country as rapidly as possible.

I found my brother, who had been on circuit when the war began, and could not get back to his home at Kimberley. He had been for some time at the Cape, and was shortly going to England.

I met a good many friends in Cape Town; some from Kimberley who had come down to recruit after the siege. All the civilians whom I met from there were loud in their appreciation of Mr. Cecil Rhodes and the way he had worked for them and cheered them through the siege—his especial thoughtfulness for the women and children.

I took the sisters to see his beautiful house, Groot Schuur, and to tea with some old friends of mine at Kenilworth.

I was anxious to see all I could of the military hospitals and how they were managed, as I had had no experience of work for the army; but my first visit to a large Military General Hospital was not encouraging, as I thought the wards looked dirty and untidy to a degree; the men had portions of food left on their lockers from previous meals, and this food was covered with flies. Knowing how much enteric there was in the camp, this, I thought, a great source of danger. The men were cheery, as usual, but complained that sleep was difficult to obtain owing to the live-stock in the beds; in some of the wards the legs of the beds were placed in condensed milk tins (containing some disinfectant), but even this was not always successful.

Another day I visited the Portland Hospital, and found everything very trim and the men very comfortable; the sisters had very nice quarters; they seemed rather horrified to hear that we had not brought any English maids with us, as they said they could never get on without theirs in this savage land (four miles from Cape Town!); but I have had to do with servants out here before, and prefer to manage with natives.

I subsequently visited another large general hospital, and found it much better kept than the first one, and the patients more comfortable; so I conclude it depends on the head a good deal, and not so much on the system.

A party of wounded men came in while I was there, most of them convalescents, but a few looked rather bad, and it seemed to be a very long time before they were put to bed.

I also visited the Red Cross Depot, and saw a good many ladies at work packing bags for the ambulance trains—a suit of pyjamas, a sponge, a handkerchief, a little writing-paper and a pencil, &c., in each bag, which must be a most welcome present for a soldier straight from the veldt.

We re-embarked on the same ship on 24th March, and had a very rough trip up the coast, calling at Port Elizabeth and East London. At the latter place the weather was very hot with a cloudy sky, and all the officers were in their white suits, when we were suddenly *struck* by a tremendous rain-storm with thunder and lightning, and the wind howling in the rigging; they had no time to change out of their white clothes, and in a few minutes looked like drowned rats.

The steam was up and everything made fast in case we should have to put out to sea, but the storm soon passed over.

We reached Durban on 31st March, and now there is much speculation as to where we are to pitch our camp.

XXVII

When we arrived at Durban the town was very full, and the sisters had to stay on board until rooms could be found for them in a boarding-house. Late in the afternoon a tug came out with a message that we were to disembark and go to a house called "Sea Breeze" in Smith Street. It was rather rough at the anchorage, and we had to get into a basket and were slung over the ship's side into the tug, then the tug had to go round and pick up a lot of lighters that had been supplying other ships with coal, &c., and by the time we got into harbour it was getting dusk, and the Customs House, supposing that all the passengers had landed earlier, was closed.

I had meant to leave our heavy baggage in the Customs House till we knew where we were going; but it was impossible to leave it loose on the jetty, and there were no cabs or trolleys about, but a mob of riksha boys, dressed up in feathers and horns and beads (and very little else), who were all clamouring to be allowed to transport us up town. Eventually we piled our baggage on these rikshas, and, distributing the sisters amongst it, we gave the boys the address, and, with much shouting, our cavalcade started off at a trot; we soon reached Smith Street, but then our troubles began, no one knowing Sea Breeze; we searched up and down the street, and one old gentleman told me he had lived all his life in Smith Street, but had never seen a Sea Breeze there!

I tried all the places where I thought our officers might be—the R.A.M.C. Depot, hotels, &c.—but could not find them, the sisters all very tired and hungry, and some of them rather nervous; then, by good luck, we met our Major, who had come out to see if we were comfortable in our quarters, and discovered that we had been given the name of the wrong street!

About 9 P.M. we found the house; but the landlady had given us up, and, thinking we should not land till the morning, had gone out; but some other lodgers (refugees from Johannesburg) raided the larder for our benefit, and we thoroughly enjoyed our supper.

The next day we found the idea had been to send us up to Mooi River, but it was thought that, with the winter coming on, that would be a cold place for sick troops, so we had better be nearer the coast; and then a Durban gentleman came forward, and most kindly offered the use of his estate of 150 acres at Pinetown; it is only about seventeen miles from Durban, but much higher up and more healthy; so the offer was gratefully accepted, and the building was at once begun.

Then followed a time when we all had to forget that we had come out to "nurse the sick and wounded," and turn to work at other jobs.

Before they were ready for us to go up to Pinetown we were all inoculated against typhoid. It was not a pleasant experience: my temperature went up to 102°, and I had intense abdominal pain and headache; it seemed like a very concentrated touch of typhoid, but it kept us in bed only two or three days, and the following five or six days we felt as weak as though we had been ill for a month.

As soon as possible I went up to see where our hospital was to be built, and found them busy levelling the ground for the tin pavilions.

There were three permanent buildings already up on the land; one, we thought, would make a good ward for officers (eight beds); another had a large room we thought would do for our staff mess-room, and some small rooms suitable for medical officers' bedrooms; and the third was a row of rooms that was apportioned for sisters' rooms, and various offices, stores, &c.

The orderlies were established in tents a little way off; they were all St. John's Ambulance men, and camping out was a new experience for them, so of course they did not know how to make themselves as comfortable as regular soldiers would have done in a new camp. They had joined expecting to have the excitement of stretcher work at the front, and when they were told off to level the ground for the buildings, or to carry up the planks and the heavy boxes from the railway trucks, and to help the builders put up the pavilions, there was a good deal of grumbling.

At first the Major in command would not hear of our going up to stay until they had got some more of the stores up—beds, sheets, &c.; but when he found how slowly they got on, and how discontented the men were at having to rough it, he gave leave for me to go up with one other sister, as we thought we might help a bit, and, at any rate, could show the men we were willing to take our share.

The hospital we had brought out was for one hundred beds, but there was urgent need for more beds, so the P.M.O. had given orders that more huts were to be sent to us, and that we were to open as a two hundred bed hospital.

The railway was so hard worked that we had the greatest difficulty to get trucks to bring the building materials up from Durban, and the docks at Durban were so crowded with stores that it was most difficult to get the things through.

Some of our medical officers worked nobly at the docks, getting the things packed on to trucks, while the others superintended the unloading at Pinetown.

Every engine seemed to be needed for taking men, horses, stores, water, &c., up to the front, and the only wonder was that so few accidents occurred on the much over-worked single line of rails.

We had landed on the last day of March, and on the evening of 12th April Sister —— and I went up to Pinetown by rail, taking all the sisters' heavy baggage; and the other sisters went to give some temporary help on one of the hospital ships at Durban, until we could fix up some rooms for them. Some of the officers met us at the station, and a fatigue party had brought a truck for our baggage. A tramp of about ten minutes through thick sand brought us to our new abode.

Our first meal, a kind of supper, was somewhat quaint; a bare deal table in a room dimly lighted by two candles stuck into bottles; plates, knives, and forks had to be used with great economy, as there were not enough to go round; some good salt beef and biscuits and some fruit—and we were waited upon by an orderly in his shirt sleeves, who was an engine-driver when at home in England, and knew more about greasing engines than about cleaning the grease off plates!

The weather was very hot, and the officers all looked dead tired, so we soon decided to turn in, and were escorted to our room (in the other building) by the light of a guttering candle, as there were said to be many snakes about.

They had found us two beds, and actually some sheets, but absolutely nothing else in our room. However, I hunted up the cook, and he lent me a bucket with some water in, so that we might start fair with a wash in the morning.

The next morning we were up before six, and started work in earnest, unpacking cases, sorting stores, and putting them away in different store-rooms, and trying to find the things we were most in need of for household use.

Some of the hospital fittings had been put ashore at Cape Town and not yet sent on, and more of the necessaries were still down at Durban, so that it was very difficult to push on the building work; and all the time we knew the Field Hospitals were crowded up, and needing to send men down to us to give them a chance of recovery; and we heard that the generals said they could not fight any more till they could clear the Field Hospitals.

All the cases of stores were numbered, so that when we wanted any particular thing, we had to look up in the list the number of its case, and then hunt about till we found that number; all day long it was "Have you seen 4507?"—"No, I want 5470." Sometimes we found a lot of jugs, and then could not find the basins; sometimes a lot of saucers, and no cups; and it seemed as though we never should get order out of the chaos.

At first we had no house-boys, and the orderlies were all busy carrying the building materials up, so Sister and I kept the bedrooms tidy, and the medical officers (in return) carried the water for the baths! As soon as I could, I annexed a fine old Kaffir as a house-boy, and "John" is a great stand-by now.

We tried first of all to fit up rooms with the bare necessary furniture for the rest of the officers and sisters, so that they could all come up and help us.

If you saw the jetty at Durban you would wonder that any stores ever got sent up to their right destination; literally hundreds of tons of boxes stacked up in hopeless confusion. Durban is a bit overdone by military requirements, and quite run out of some stores.

On April 3rd we were made very anxious by a strong rumour that Mafeking had fallen. They say that *all* the little children have died there. Yesterday we heard of the loss of a British convoy and five guns, and also that the Boers were going into laager again quite near to where Cronje was taken.

Durban is full of refugees, and of Ladysmith people recruiting after the siege. I went over one of the hospital ships, the *Lismore Castle*, before I came up here, and it was melancholy to see the *skeletons* from Ladysmith; one quite young fellow told me he had come here from India, got typhoid soon after the siege began, then, as soon as he began to convalesce, the only food they could give him was mealy meal and a little horse-flesh, so he got dysentery. He is now mending, but it is slow work with them all.

Before we came, our rooms had been occupied by refugees, and fleas abound; I catch about six *ter die* and once in the night. Luckily we are fairly free from mosquitoes. It is awfully hot, and the medical officers go about in trousers and vests only: we wish we could wear as little!

This is a very scrappy letter; we work from 6 A.M. to dusk, and then I have been scribbling a little before turning in, but I am weary to a degree, and must fill up the gaps in my next.

XXVIII

You must not expect me to tell you anything about the progress of the war; the papers here give us very little news; of course we are constantly hearing many startling rumours, but they are frequently contradicted the next day, and probably you have more reliable news of the doings of our troops in your papers at home than we have.

So I will just jot down things about our daily work here.

We are getting into order by degrees, but at present life is rather a struggle against difficulties.

You see we are not quite a Civil Hospital, nor are we quite a Military Hospital; for the 100 beds we brought out we were well equipped, and had many more comforts than a Military Hospital would have been provided with, but now we are to have 200 beds, and our resources are somewhat strained.

I found that the mess waiter was in his shirt sleeves because the poor man had been nursing a case of scarlet fever on board ship, and all his kit had to be burnt, so I fitted him up in some pyjama coats to wait at table, until I could get time to go in to Durban and buy him some white drill jackets.

After a few days' work at unpacking, we got quite civilised in our room fittings, and sent for the other sisters to come up and help.

If there had not been such need for hurry in getting the place ready, it would really have been very amusing; much of the furniture had been a good deal damaged on the way, and we all tried our hands at mending—to see our senior surgeon (who is on the staff of a large hospital in England) sitting on the ground trying to fit a leg on to a washstand, or to make a drawer run into a chest of drawers, is a fine sight; I have taken a few snaps with my kodak of the staff in unprofessional garb, and doing unprofessional jobs. I hope they will come out all right, but I don't see much prospect of having time to develop them.

The theatre is fitted up, but has not been used yet, and Mr. —— is working hard getting the X-Ray room into order, and his apparatus fixed up.

Our food supplies (always called "skoff" here—the Kaffirs' name for food) were very erratic at first. Sometimes no meat would turn up, and then we made shift with bully-beef, which is really quite good, or sardines; sometimes no bread, then we used the barrel of biscuits that lived in the mess-room—you have no idea how difficult it is to eat enough of those biscuits to satisfy you (they are nearly as hard as dog biscuits!), and in about half-an-hour you feel starving again; sometimes there is no butter— then marmalade. Now things are coming up more regularly, and I hope they will continue to do so, as it is easy for us to joke about short commons for ourselves, but it is no joke when you have sick men needing careful feeding up.

One thing is very nice, and that is that the fruit is nearly ripe, and we shall soon have plenty of pineapples and oranges.

Our cook seems to try to make the best of things; he is only quite a lad, but he is managing to cook for us all (including the men), with only wood under a sort of gridiron, in the open air.

There was much joy the other day when we came across a case of "Mother's Crushed Oats"! and nearly all seem to enjoy porridge for breakfast. As it is still very hot, the food supplies are difficult to manage, the meat hardly keeping from one meal to another, even when cooked; and with very limited store-rooms I find it very difficult to see that everything is kept covered up and fly-proof.

So far we have had no fresh milk, but now two cows have arrived, and I am having to watch the boys milk them, as we pay for the milk by the number of bottles supplied!

We have just heard that the poor old *Mexican* has gone down on her voyage out: no lives lost, but we fear our letters have gone to the bottom with her.

One thing I am worried about is that a big tank I had especially asked to have, in which we might boil all the typhoid linen, has been broken on the way, and I don't think I shall be able to get another. We are establishing a place for the washerwomen behind the hospital, on a slope where their water will run away from our direction; I should like to have had a separate place for the staff's washing, but cannot manage it, so must be contented with keeping special women and special tubs, &c., for it.

The men are really working very well now, and it is hard work they have to do; they required a good deal of persuasion to work on Saturday afternoon; but we hear the Field Hospitals are crowded up with 2000 sick, on this side alone, so we must push on the building.

We are getting everything into order in the big store-room, so that as soon as any of the big pavilions are finished we shall have all the fittings quite ready to issue.

I have been down to see the P.M.O. in Durban. He seems very nice, and willing to give us all the help he can; he seems glad that we are going to have the extra beds, and promises to send us more doctors, sisters, and orderlies; we rather hope that some of the orderlies will be R.A.M.C. men, and that they will put a little backbone into our crew, who, I daresay, will be better when we get into order, but many of them are now rather inclined to say "We didn't pass our exams, and come out here, to do navvies' work."

Of course I shall be glad to have the larger place, as I know it is so badly needed, but the prospect of seeing 100 sick men properly looked after by these untrained men was alarming, and now the prospect of 200 sick men with more (possibly) untrained orderlies, plus some unknown sisters, is more alarming still; but I suppose we shall shake along somehow.

I shall be so glad when the men can get time to cut the long grass round the camp, as there are a good many snakes about (two have been killed quite near my room). We all wear canvas gaiters, as a sort of protection; but there are other weird creatures about, and one night a wire came from the next station to say that a leopard, or some such creature, had carried off a Kaffir baby, and we were to look out for the beast; so the men were much excited, but they have not seen anything of him.

Last Sunday was Easter Sunday, and the men had a much needed day of rest, but the sisters and officers went on most of the day unpacking and sorting the things most urgently needed. We knocked off in the evening, and went to service at the Pinetown church.

The next day (April 16th) we had started work as usual, when the Sergeant-major's whistle summoned all hands: a wire had come to say that a troop train had been thrown off the line about three miles from here.

The Major went off with the medical officers and orderlies, with stretchers. I provided them with brandy, water, a mug, a corkscrew, &c., and then hunted up some lint and bandages, and a few splints, and sent them after them.

Two or three orderlies who were sick in camp came down to see what the alarm meant, and wanted to go to help, but they did not look fit for a three miles' run in the burning sun, so I told them to collect all the natives who were left behind, and we made a hasty clearance of the building that was to be an officers' ward (temporarily used as a store-room). We set several boys to work to scrub the floor and clean the windows, while the orderlies fitted some beds together, and the sisters collected the bedding and made them up, and I got the most necessary ward fittings out of the store, so that when the stretcher party arrived we had quite a workable little surgical ward ready for them.

Two poor fellows had been killed, and fifteen mules were either dead or had to be shot; three men of the Army Service Corps were injured, one with a badly broken leg, and the others with concussion, &c., and two black mule-drivers had each a dreadfully smashed up arm. The Major had a tent pitched for these natives, not far from the ward. It is a wonder they were not killed, as they were in the same truck with the poor mules.

One sister and some orderlies were told off to look after these, our first, patients; and then we returned to our building occupations.

I did not put a night sister on for these few cases, but I take a prowl round some time during the night (the fleas always wake me up at least once, otherwise I am so tired I don't think I could wake myself), just to see that the orderlies are awake, and managing all right, and the medical officers go round the last thing before turning in, and we are all about by 6 A.M.

One of the injured A.S.C. men had been ill before he arrived here, and it looks as though he is in for typhoid.

Last night, after a more than usually scorching day, we had torrents of rain. The poor orderlies were washed out of their tents, and all their things were soaked. They are not used to roughing it, and don't enjoy it.

It seems ever so long since I came up here, but I had been here only four days before these cases came in, and we hope in about another week to be able to send word that we are ready to receive patients from the front.

XXIX

PINETOWN, NATAL,
May 1900.

Now we are really at work at last, and though I can't say everything is working very smoothly, I think the patients are being well looked after, and I suppose we must expect to have to worry through difficulties for some time to come.

On April 26th the Princess Christian Hospital train brought us fourteen officers and sixteen men, all stretcher cases, and all very ill.

They had come from Field Hospitals, and if one did not know how impossible it is to nurse them or even feed them up there, one would say it was almost murder to have sent them a journey of many hours (over 200 miles) in a jolting train.

There were no wounded in this first batch, and I think only about four or five who were not suffering from typhoid in one stage or another, from a few days, up to three weeks or more.

It was day and night work for us for the first two or three days, as each man seemed to need individual nursing if he was to have a chance of pulling round; the orderlies (though very willing) had everything to learn of ward duties; they could not even undress these men when they had been lifted on to their beds, much less had they any idea of washing them; a delirious man was a new experience to them, and if he got out of bed and lay on the floor, the orderly would go and ask Sister what he had better do!

The doctors told us that four of these patients could not live through the first night (several of them had severe hæmorrhage), but they all struggled through that night, and it was a week later when one poor fellow of the Royal Artillery slipped through our fingers from sheer exhaustion, without ever having become conscious. His mates told us that he had been in a hospital previously with a sunstroke, and had been down with typhoid for some time before he arrived here.

I can't describe the condition of these men; they have not had their clothes off for weeks, creeping things are numerous, but we are getting them clean by degrees. Those who have been ill some time have sore backs—I can't say "*bed*-sores," as they have had no beds.

Many of them have come from Elandslaagte, and I believe they are very short of both milk and water up there—none of the latter for washing purposes.

Several of the men had been with us over a week before they became conscious of their surroundings at all; but in the case of those who *were* conscious, the comforts of a good bed, and a good wash, brought tears of gratitude to their eyes. With many of them it was months since they had slept in a bed: few have done so since they landed in this country, and some of them seem such boys to have gone through so much.

I spent a good deal of my time at first helping the sister in the officers' ward, getting her patients washed and made comfortable, and it was most piteous to see these young fellows—most of them, probably, brought up in luxury—so wasted and thin, and *so* grateful for the little that we could spare time to do for their comfort.

Lieutenant —— had been laid up for two months with a bullet in the groin, and is now very ill again with typhoid.

Captain ——, of the R.A.M.C., had been all through the siege of Ladysmith, and had typhoid up there; now he has liver trouble and looks wretchedly ill; I fancy he will have to go home for operation.

Captain ——, of the Royal Artillery, was the worst case of typhoid amongst the officers, for some time his temperature persisting in keeping up to 105 and 106, and he was very delirious; he was always thinking he could see parties of Boers, and he told me I was the worst scout he had ever come across, as I did not see them. He is doing well now.

Lieutenant ——, of the Army Service Corps, had been ill for four weeks with typhoid before he was landed here (still with a very high temperature).

He told me that no less than five times had he been moved on a stretcher, from one place to another, as his regiment shifted about, and he said that the order to move always seemed to come in the evening, when his temperature was at its highest, and he was feeling so bad, that at last he begged them to leave him behind to die; they had never been able to give him suitable food, and often not enough of unsuitable, and when at last he got to the line he had 280 miles of jolting over a single-line rail, before he reached us—such treatment for a case that, at home, we should be almost afraid to lift from one bed to another! But he is really mending now, and I hope we shall soon be able to send him home to recruit.

I have never had to give so much stimulant to any patients as we have had to give to these men; all the first night I was going round giving milk and brandy, or bovril, to the worst cases, while the night sister sponged those whose temperatures were the highest; several of the men were on ten ounces of brandy for the first few days. They have been so overworked, and underfed, for some months past that they did not seem to have an ounce of strength left to battle with the fever.

An Army Lady Superintendent is supposed to take charge of a ward herself —generally the officers' ward; but I have not taken a ward yet, as, until we fill up, there are enough sisters, and it seems more profitable for me to go round supplying the sisters' needs from the stores, looking after the cooking, and the house-boys, and the washerwomen (I fear that my hair will turn grey in my efforts to keep the typhoid linen separate), to say nothing of the cows, which are not a success; and we have had to resort to frozen milk from Australia—generally good, but sometimes there is a difficulty about unfreezing it.

We have no Quartermaster here, and the man in charge of the stores is quite unused to his job, so I have to see to a great many things with which an Army Lady Superintendent has, as a rule, nothing to do.

I am very much afraid some of our orderlies will be getting typhoid; of course they find it difficult to realise a danger they can't see, and though we all lecture them about taking precautions, we are so busy ourselves, that it is difficult to enforce them; and just at first there were so many patients quite unconscious and with severe diarrhœa and hæmorrhage, so that it meant constant changing of sheets, &c., by the orderlies.

I think I told you some of the orderlies were ill when our first patients (from the train accident) arrived; it proved to be a form of dengue fever they had, and now the medical officers also are indulging in it; it is rather like influenza—high fever for two or three days, and then they are very weak and pulled down for a few more days. I only hope the sisters will refrain from having it until the orderlies have had a little more education: at present they are about as useful as an average ward-maid at home, and the sisters have to act as sister, staff nurse, and probationer too; but I don't want to grumble at them as they are working well, anxious to learn, and very patient with the men (some of them half delirious) who call "Orderly, orderly" all day long.

If they had had a few R.A.M.C. men amongst them, or even one or two R.A.M.C. ward-masters, it would have been easier; as it is, there is not a single man amongst them who knows anything of the usual routine in a hospital, though they are well up in "First Aid" (for which we have no use here).

The buildings are getting on, and we are ready for more patients as soon as they can get a train to bring them down. We hear nothing of more medical officers, sisters, or orderlies as yet.

One of the men said to me that he did not think any of us could understand what a luxury it was to have a wash, a comfortable bed, and clean clothes; that for months he had been marching and sleeping (in the open) in one suit of clothes, frequently wet through, and remaining wet until the sun came out to dry them; he said that on the high veldt the nights were very cold, and they frequently had nothing but their greatcoats to sleep in; if they were lucky, and the baggage waggons had kept up with them, they would also have a blanket and perhaps a mackintosh sheet; but that the baggage waggons had a habit of getting stuck at the last drift, and then they had only what they carried.

If we had only come out to South Africa to nurse this one batch of thirty officers and men back to health, I think it would have been worth while, for they were just about as bad as they well could be, and one can't help thinking of the anxiety of their poor friends at home, who will have seen them reported on the "danger lists" from their Field Hospitals; and we go plodding on night and day trying to make them pull round. Only one man has died, and I think the rest will get on, though some of them are still pretty bad.

Captain —— had Cheyne Stokes breathing for two nights, and made us very anxious, but now he is distinctly better.

The Bishop of Pretoria came to lunch with us the other day, and was very nice in visiting the men.

We are expecting more men any day now, and on the 25th of this month we are to be officially "opened" (on Princess Christian's birthday, I believe); a crowd of people are expected from Durban and from Pietermaritzburg.

I could not help thinking the other day, when all these thirty men were dumped in upon us in a couple of hours, of the old days in London when we thought we had had a very heavy day if six or eight patients were admitted to our ward in a day; and there we had everything ready to hand, and several well-drilled nurses to help. Here I can see it will take a little time before the sisters will realise that it is useless to try to have things done just the same as we can at home, and for them to distinguish between the *essentials* of good nursing, which we must have, and the superfluous finish, which we must do without.

XXX

We have had a stiff time of work since I wrote last. I think I told you that several orderlies were ill, when our first cases came in, with dengue fever, and soon the medical officers began knocking up with it—first one and then another; next, the sisters took it; no one has been very ill, but the fever was high for several days, and, of course, they were weak and seedy after it went down; so we have not had a full staff at work for some time, and with lots of bad cases in the wards it has made things very difficult.

Several odd cases have been straying in, and on the 17th we took in five officers, and then on the 19th of last month we admitted eight officers and thirty men from Modder Spruit, most of them very ill, and one poor fellow so bad with hæmorrhage (enteric) that he died the same night.

We had to open a second officers' ward, and the sister put in charge was very hopeless (at having so many bad cases, and such inefficient help); so I had to spend a good deal of time helping her look after the worst cases, and then the next morning after they arrived I found she had dengue fever and could not come on duty; so I had to take charge of her ward for a few days, and do the best I could in looking after the patients with the help of the orderlies, amidst constant interruptions and appeals for help or advice from different parts of the camp.

With every one so new to the work—the cook quite unused to military ways or the serving of hospital diets, the storekeeper hardly knowing where anything is, or whether he ought to issue it when he did know, ten Kaffir women washing who could not read the marks on the linen, and so were quite incapable of returning it to the right place without my assistance, and, to do the house work, several new Kaffir boys who really are quite "raw" and want constant looking after (they rejoice in the names of John, Monday, Charlie, and Cup-of-tea; they can speak about six words of English between them, and it is awfully funny hearing the orderlies trying to make them understand), with much other work needing to be done in connection with fitting up new wards and preparing for our opening day ceremony—you can imagine it was difficult to be tied up in one ward with a lot of sick officers who required one's best attention, and more; but it had to be done, and I had to leave the rest to do the best they could, only going round to attend to the most necessary things when I could spare half-an-hour in the day, and after the night sister came on at night.

My worst case was poor Captain ——, of the —— Dragoons, who was desperately bad from the day he came in, and was delirious most of the time; Lieutenant ——, of the same regiment (a friend of his), was very good in sitting with him for part of the day, and when he was at his worst one of the other sisters and I took turns of acting night special (as the night sister could not possibly stay with him much); but he had been thoroughly worn out with the hardships of the campaign before he got the fever, and though he lingered on so that we kept hoping he would pull through, he died on the 30th of May—our first death amongst the officers, and we all felt very sad. It was terrible for Lieutenant —— (ill with rheumatism), as he knows the captain's relations, and has been cabling to them daily. The funeral was the next day, and the station-master kindly stopped a goods train here, so that the few officer patients who were well enough might go to Pinetown to attend, and all the medical officers who could leave also went. I was too busy to go, but I helped Lieutenant —— to make a cross of white flowers to put on the coffin.

A thing that always makes me feel creepy when I am working in the store is the sight, in one corner, of a little pile of coffins that have been sent up from Durban; of course it is really necessary to keep them ready as, in this climate, the funeral must be the day following the death, but we have had them covered up now, as I did not like the men to see them when they went up to the store for things.

All that last batch of men were frightfully poisoned with enteric, and nothing seemed to stop it; six of them have died, and most of them had symptoms of blood poisoning too.

I don't think I told you that the two sisters who went to help on one of the hospital ships till we could get rooms ready for them, came up at the beginning of May. They brought a poor account of the nursing on that particular ship, and said that, when they went away, there was no fully-trained nurse left on board; that a large proportion of the men who had been ill any length of time, had sore backs (some before they reached the ship). It seems sad that when there are so many fully-trained nurses in England longing to come out, these poor fellows should not be getting the best nursing they might have, even right down at the base.

On the 21st of May we heard that Mafeking was really relieved, and on the 25th of May we were officially "opened." General Wolfe Murray was to have performed the ceremony, but he could not come, as General Buller had sent for him, so the Bishop of Natal and Colonel Morris did it between them.

There were special trains from Maritzburg and Durban; a good many people to lunch, and such a crowd in the afternoon—no one seems to know how many, but I think we gave tea to about five hundred. Fortunately, Sister —— was on duty again, so I was not fixed up in her ward, but she was still needing help with her bad cases. I made the teabags in the middle of the night while I took my turn at sitting by poor Captain ——, and several people who live near here were very kind in helping me arrange flowers on the day, and they cut up cake for me. We had a lot of coolie waiters up from Durban, and our house-boys and some whom Mrs. T. (a most kindly neighbour) sent to help, were washing up all the afternoon.

I can't say I enjoyed the day, as we had several patients very ill, and two poor fellows died that day, but we managed to keep their ward (and one of the officers' wards) closed to visitors, so they were not disturbed, and everything went smoothly and well.

When the visitors were leaving, I asked the Major if the orderlies might come and finish up the cakes, &c., as there was some good tea in the urns still, and they had all been working very well, so he told the sergeant-major they might. I was rather amused at one thing: I took a big tin and gave it to the sergeant-major, asking him to save a few cakes for the night orderlies, but he pointed out to me they were all present; the news of a tea and some good "skoff" had brought them all down from their tents, and they soon made short work of the remains.

I went into Durban one day to do some necessary shopping, and on the train met Colonel Galway, the P.M.O., going down to inspect the hospital ships. He was very nice to me, and told me that if I liked to engage any more sisters out here I might do so, and he would take them on; so I am engaging a lady as a kind of probationer and housekeeper. Her husband is at the front, and she wants to help, and I think she will be able to relieve me a good deal by looking after the house-boys, putting out linen, &c.

Our sisters are working awfully well, but some of them don't get on well with the orderlies—a great mistake: they don't seem able to hide the fact that they think the orderlies very useless and incapable, and consequently the orderlies don't do their best in working with them; it is a great pity, as the men are quite willing and anxious to learn, and are very patient in having to do many jobs that must be very trying to them.

At last I have got a nice white woman to look after the Kaffir washing ladies, and she will do the starching, &c., for the staff. Two of the Kaffirs were washing all day with babies tied on their backs—such jolly fat and shiny little black-a-moors. I gave them an empty packing-case with some sawdust in it and a mat, and both the babies and mothers were delighted.

I actually had a ride the other day; Mrs. D. kindly lent me a horse, and I rode with the Major over to a most interesting Trappist monastery. The Trappist Fathers cultivate a lot of land, and teach the native boys various trades. They are going to supply us with eggs, vegetables, &c., and the Major arranged with them that they should visit our Roman Catholic patients, and, if any of them die, they will bury them in their churchyard.

We shall have to have a horse for funeral purposes, and we have been offered a rather nice-looking black animal, so I hope that, to my varied duties, will be added that of keeping the funeral horse exercised!

I don't care much for walking about here, there is so much long grass, and you get covered with ticks (to say nothing of one's natural fear of snakes), so an occasional hour or two on horseback will be refreshing, though up to now I have hardly left the camp except to go to church at Pinetown once on Sundays.

I had a letter the other day from the Secretary of the Durban Ladies' Club to say they had made us all honorary members—a very kind and friendly attention on their part. It is a nice club, but whether we shall ever have time to make use of it remains to be proved.

There are many strange animals about here: a huge owl is getting quite tame, and comes to be fed by the night sister.

The men are trying to shoot a wild cat, but can't get up near to it. After hearing them talking about it, I was rather frightened the other night (sleeping with my door and window open), when something jumped from the window on to my bed; I felt it creeping towards me, and was just going to dive under the bedclothes when it began to purr, and I found it was the camp kitten!

XXXI

It is rather difficult to know what to write about that will interest you. There is always plenty of work, but it is not of an exciting nature—just steady plodding on, with difficulties always cropping up and having to be waded through.

If one had time to sit and talk to the patients one could hear many exciting tales, but most of my time is spent with those who are too ill for much conversation. I think I told you of the arrival of the officers and men from Modder Spruit. Opening the large ward for these officers caused some difficulty, as it is such a long way from the kitchen, but we soon got up from Durban some hot tins, covers, &c., and the feeding is going better now.

Major —— had been very ill with ptomaine poisoning before he arrived here. He has been a difficult case to feed in this climate, and has been very slow in getting up any strength; but he is well on the mend now. Then there was a bright-faced *boy* with acute rheumatism, who said he had not been in bed for six months, and it was "just heavenly." Lieutenant —— (a bishop's son) is 6 ft. 6 in., and we have to wrap up his feet on a chair beyond the end of his bed. He has enteric, but not so very badly; he called me to him the other day, and told me that he had had the most bitter disappointment of his life—the doctor had ordered him an egg, and he waited patiently till tea-time, expecting a nice boiled egg, but he never knew the orderly would bring him a beaten-up egg, and he had nearly drunk it before he recognised it!

Then there is Second-Lieutenant ——, who looks about sixteen, and who only joined his regiment nine months ago, but he has seen a lot of fighting, and was at Spion Kop, Pieter's Hill, and other battles. Some of his men are here, and they think a great deal of him; they say at Spion Kop all his seniors were either killed or wounded, but he led the men on as calmly and well as possible; I believe he got a "mention" for it. His captain wrote to me so nicely asking after him, and said, "He is a good boy, and A1 when the bullets are flying." He had been wounded badly, and now has enteric, but only slightly. The other officers all call him "the boy." I hope we shall be able to send him home to his people soon, as I think he has done his share.

Some of these officers are beginning to get about now, and they *will* go to visit the officers in the small ward and persuade them to give them tea there, and then return and get their own tea as well. They say they are "making up for past hardships"! Amongst that same batch of men there were two or three rather smart R.A.M.C. men, and we don't think they are going to be fit for duty at the front again this campaign: they will be quite contented to stay here, and work as soon as they are well enough.

We have just got the electric light into working order; and, though it is rather erratic, and often goes out, on the whole it is a great comfort.

There has been a case of bubonic plague in Durban, but they don't seem to think it is likely to spread.

Twenty more orderlies have arrived, St. John's Ambulance men, and the buildings were all complete by the end of May.

I have had a few rides on the funeral horse, and, as it is very tame in harness, I was astonished to find it was quite gay and hard to hold; but we have found out that it was once a racehorse, and of course it has never had a side-saddle on before.

Our nice compounder has been awfully ill with appendicitis and dysentery. We have had to write each mail to his people, but now I am glad to say he is doing well. Several of the orderlies are down with enteric, including our mess-room waiter; so "Cup-of-tea" has to wait on our mess of eighteen, and needs a good deal of looking after.

I expect they will give me another orderly soon, but so many are ill, and the wards are heavy, and need a good many men for night duty. Every few nights the orderlies have to do a spell on night (as well as their ordinary day) duty, so they are rather inclined to grumble, and it is difficult for them to keep awake; but I don't think any of them do longer hours than I do, as I prowl about a good deal in the night when the cases first come down and are bad; so they don't grumble too loud.

The sisters seemed to be getting rather fagged out, so I have begun to give them in turn a monthly day off, and I look after their wards. I find it is rather useful, as I get a good opportunity of seeing how they have managed, and also of learning how much the orderlies are good for; it is quite touching how good they are to me: they want to show me they can be trusted, and they do everything they possibly can to save me trouble on these "days off." From the sergeant-major downwards they have always been very nice to me, and I am sure I do very little for them (except when they are ill and need fussing over) beyond scolding them for misdeeds for which the sisters report them.

I wonder whether they guess that, all the time, I feel that the sisters are expecting too much of them!

I was amused when a new sergeant arrived with twenty men the other day; of course, at first they did not know any of us, and when I met them and said "Good morning," they simply gaped. The next day I had a fatigue party sent up to tidy the china and linen store; of course our old batch of men saluted when I went to show them what I wanted done; and I expect the new men received a few words from them on their slack manners afterwards, for since then there has been a very stiff draw up and salute whenever they come for orders or with a message. I hear the army sisters are not saluted as a rule.

I think I told you how much we suffered from fleas at first; now they are quite banished. We have twenty coolies, and a good orderly in charge of them, and they do all the sanitary work, and sweep and scrub and generally keep the place tidy (they also have to dig the graves), and since we have got rid of all the packing-cases, and everything is trim and tidy, the fleas have disappeared.

So far we have had very few wounded in—nearly all enteric or dysentery, with some cases of camp fever, rheumatism, &c.; the medical officers are disappointed at so little surgical work, but I don't think I mind, as we can feel we are actually saving the lives of some of these men by sheer hard nursing, and that is good enough for me; sometimes a man sees that I am worrying about a patient who does not seem to be improving, or who is going downhill, and he will come up and say "Never mind, Sister, he would have been dead long ago if he had been left in that Field Hospital any longer; you have given the chap a chance." It is grand to see the first batch of men, who came to us so desperately ill, so haggard, starved, dirty, and miserable, getting about now in their blue suits, looking so clean and bright, though still very thin.

Some of them are beginning to need to be amused, and the knitting wool and materials for worsted work that I brought out are coming in very useful; in fact, they will soon be finished, but the Durban ladies have kindly promised to send me more.

Several of the men were making worsted belts in one ward the other day, and a big Scotchman looked in and asked them to go for a walk, but they refused, saying they were busy, and the Scotchman was heard to mutter "They've all turned blooming milliners!"

Lieutenant —— (the giant) is getting on very well, and he was always saying I must stay and amuse him, or else give him some toys, so I have started him with some worsted work, and he is more contented, and as fussy about my providing him with the right shades of wool as any old lady. The Lieutenant in the next bed has learnt to knit, and Major ——, the ptomaine poisoning case, looks surprised at their babyishness.

The other day Sister B. was going to have a day off, and these boys, overhearing her instructions about themselves, made up some poetry on the subject (which I enclose), and Sister won't hear the last of it for some time.

We have a service in the wards every other Sunday, and the hymn-books I brought out are most useful.

June 13.—The last few days have been very busy and very sad.

On the 7th we had a trainload of patients—two officers and seventy-three men—several of the men very bad. I was up most of the first night helping with the bad cases, but one poor fellow died the next day (he was never conscious after he got here); that day also, Sister —— knocked up with slight fever, so I had to take over her ward, and there were several bad cases in it.

The orderlies are knocking up with enteric—six of them warded; and I have hardly liked to leave them at night, as several of them are inclined to be delirious and try to get out of bed.

L. was the worst, but he did not seem in any special danger till last Wednesday: on that day I was Orderly Sister for the afternoon, and on my first round I talked to them all, and he seemed much as usual, but on my second round I found him distinctly worse, and with a failing pulse. I called his doctor, and we tried everything possible, but he soon became unconscious, and died at 7.30 P.M. All the orderlies are dreadfully cut up; several of them come from the same place in Yorks. He was such a fine, strong young fellow, and it seems only the other day that he was acting as groom, and put me up on the black pony, and was so pleased I could manage him. He was a butcher by trade, rough in his ways, but so good-natured; I must write to his poor mother.

He had a military funeral, and we let every orderly go who could be spared. The clergyman asked me if the men would like to have a hymn in church, so we sang "Brief life is here our portion." Several people sent wreaths, and the men are going to make a wooden cross. This was the first death amongst our staff. Having so many orderlies ill, and the place pretty full, we have been very busy, and many of the men have had to do eighteen-hour shifts every two or three days: that is to say, their usual twelve-hour day and half the night. So they are having a heavy time of it. Enclosure:—

SISTER'S "DAY OFF"

There once was a Sister called Baker,
Of beds she's an excellent maker,
    She knows temperatures too,
    And between "me and you"
Is of medicines an excellent shaker.

She shows each man's vice—how to treat it,
And warns Sister H. how to meet it:
    "No. 2 you can trust
    But show T— a crust,
Well, it's a thousand to one he'll eat it."

She dilates on the treatment we need,
All our habits, our drinks, our feed;
    "I repeat, Mr. T—
    Doesn't realise all, but
He cannot be trusted for greed."

"Mr. N—, however, is wise,
At the sight of eggs hard boiled he sighs,
    D— eschew them I must
    And that beautiful crust,
For on me Sister Baker relies."

You may ask how we know what was said
The culprit there lying in bed,
    Overheard in the dark,
    The whispered remark,
And tears of hot anger he shed.

The moral is not far to seek:
A crust perforates you when weak,
    While eavesdropping at night
    Is really not right
For it's apt to raise anger and pique.

(*With apologies to the Authors.*)

XXXII

Since my last letter we have had a good many changes of patients, some being sent back to the front, and others going home by various hospital ships. It is so nice to see some who were carried in desperately ill, able to march down to the train so cheery and bright, and tremendously grateful.

We sent thirty home by the H.S. *Dunera* last month, and were just hoping to have time to breathe, and to get the sheets and blankets washed, when we had a wire to tell us to expect seventy-five more; so we had a scramble to get the beds and bedding ready for them, and they nearly filled us up; but they were not quite such a *bad* lot as our previous batches had been, and there were a good many wounded by way of a change.

We were still short-handed, so had to do a good deal of sorting of patients; turning some wards into convalescent wards, that needed only occasional visits from a sister, and no night orderlies—a sergeant patient being made responsible for good order in the ward.

Several of the orderlies are still ill: the mess-room man has had a relapse, and will not be fit for work for some time; the second compounder has also been very bad with typhoid—delirious for more than a week—but I think he will do all right now; it has been awkward, as the first compounder can only just crawl about after his spell of illness.

We have had one man awfully bad with double pneumonia after a stiff turn of typhoid. Then he got a bad abscess in the jaw, and had to have it operated on; for some days his temperature hovered between 105° and 106°, but now he is doing well, and will soon be sent home.

We have been inspected by Colonel Clery, who, unfortunately, came on the day on which we had those seventy-five men in, and before we had got them all washed or their kit put away; but he was very pleasant to me, and said he was pleased with the wards and the looks of the patients, bedding, &c.

We have also had several other distinguished visitors—Sir John Furley, Sir William Stokes, and Major Baptie of the R.A.M.C., who won his V.C. at Colenso.

We have all been very sorry to hear of the death of Colonel Forrester, who had been in charge of the Princess Christian Hospital Train, and had been here several times bringing us patients.

The four months for which this hospital was given, equipped, and maintained by private generosity, are now nearly over, and in a few days we shall have become a Government Hospital. We shall then receive our pay and various allowances from the Government; and we are now arranging to separate the mess of the sisters from that of the medical officers. I expect it will be difficult to keep our stores separately, but we shall wish to live more economically than they do. For the present we have decided to share the same cook, an Indian who has been acting as our dhobie for the last few weeks, and who, we hear, is a good cook; his wife will continue to act as our dhobie; she is such a pretty little thing, with rings in her nose and bangles on her ankles and arms.

I quite expected to be superseded by an Army Sister proper when the hospital was handed over, but the P.M.O. has asked me to "carry on" (which does not mean the same in the army as it does in Cockney land!)

The other day poor Miss H. arrived. She had started from England as soon as she heard her brother was ill here, meaning to nurse him, and I think I told you he died here (our first death amongst the officers). It was awfully sad for her. I was frightfully busy the day she came, but felt I must walk over to the cemetery with her. She is a trained nurse, and we should have been very glad of her help if she could only have arrived in time, as her brother was delirious for so long, and we had to take turns at sitting up with him for some time; but everything that could possibly be done for him was done.

They do seem to muddle things a bit; in the last few weeks we have had *seven* new sisters sent to us; we would have given anything for a few of them a couple of months ago, but now there is much less fever, and many of the beds are filled with convalescents. We had no rooms for so many sisters, so had to put up tents for them.

One day we sent off a batch of over fifty men for home, emptied several wards (putting the remaining cases into other wards), and had a general clean up; the same day we had a wire to tell us to expect seventy-two men the next evening, so we had a scramble to get the linen dry and everything ready for them. They proved to be all convalescents, and they came down thinking they were going straight on board ship for home, and of course were rather disgusted at being stopped here. The next day, having got them all settled in, and their kit stowed away, we had a wire asking us to send sixty men down to Durban the next morning for home!

So, again, there was a great bustle and inspection, and the lucky sixty having been selected had to retrieve their kit from the store and be fitted up with comforts for the voyage.

We feel sure that it was all a mistake their coming here at all, and that they ought to have gone straight on board ship. Of course it gave us an awful lot of work, and did not do them any good. We must try to see the remaining twelve get off with the next batch.

The other day fifteen new orderlies came, men of the Imperial Bearer Company (chiefly recruited from refugees and other Colonials). Some of them are quite old and bearded, and there was much puffing over their march up from the station. It is so funny to have to hurry these venerable gents round the wards when they look at me solemnly through their specs, and the Tommies are rather inclined to humbug them.

Some of our original St. John's men will have to leave soon, as their time is up, and we are letting all those go who are not very keen on the work, but, unfortunately, some of the keen ones want to go too. I am sorry to lose them, and rather blame the sisters for it.

The orderlies have been awfully nice to me; two of the best have been promoted to be sergeants. One, who has been chiefly in the officers' ward (he is a railway guard at home), has been splendidly patient with them all;

and the other is the man who has been in charge of the sanitary work and managed the coolies.

I have been having a little riding lately while the extra sisters have been here, and all the sisters in turn are having a few days' leave.

One day some people asked us to go for a picnic (riding), so we collected all the screws we could, and, making a party of twelve, we rode to a very pretty waterfall about nine miles from here, and they had arranged for tea at a quaint old farmhouse near by.

Riding back by moonlight my (funeral) horse was so keen that I could hardly hold him, so I was riding ahead with one of the men, when, hearing a shout, we hurried back and found the senior civil surgeon had had a tumble. He was not much of a horseman, and they had put him on the very quietest nag, but it had stumbled, and he came off.

He managed to ride home at a walk, though he was unconscious for a few minutes at first. He was a good deal shaken, and had to keep quiet for some days.

Another day we went to the Trappist Abbey; when we arrived, they kept us waiting some time in a room, and then a meal suddenly appeared—poached eggs, delicious brown bread, honey, fruit, tea, and tamarind wine. We were surprised, as it was early in the afternoon, but we felt obliged to accept it, and it was all very good, though I shied at the tamarind wine. Afterwards they showed us round the place.

It is really wonderful what these Trappists do for the natives, with their schools, shops for bootmaking, saddlery, tanning, ironmongery, printing, photography, &c.; but whether it does the native any real and lasting good to teach him all these things is quite another matter.

Everything seems to be running more smoothly in the hospital now, and even if the place were full of bad cases (as it was at the first), now that the orderlies are getting to know their duties, we feel that we could tackle the work without the hopeless sensation of being unable to do half enough for everybody.

We are very lucky in our Major: he is very keen to have everything well done, and one can always go to consult him in any difficulty.

XXXIII

We are now a full-blown Military Hospital, instead of being partly civil and partly military. Everybody had talked so much about the coming of "red tape" that I had been a little nervous about the change; but, except just in the transition stage, everything has gone very smoothly, and when everybody gets used to the military ways I think it will be all right. Personally, I shall have much less worry and responsibility, for we now have a Lieutenant-Quartermaster of the R.A.M.C., and I shall not have to try to look after the linen and other stores. Moreover, a batch of Indians has arrived and gone into camp, with a good headman, and they will do all the washing over which I have had so many struggles with careless Kaffir women.

I had to attend a big function down in Durban, when the residents presented the gentleman who gave this hospital with an illuminated address. There were many speeches, and much "butter" for all the staff. I was presented with a large photograph of the address.

We have had a good many changes in the staff, and among the civil surgeons who have gone home is the only one of us who understood the electric light plant, with which, in consequence, we have had difficulties. I hope we shall soon find an orderly who understands it, as, when the light fails and we have to grope about with candles, the men cannot read, and find the long evenings very dull.

I hear many interesting tales when I go about trying to amuse the men on these occasions; the other day I was called to enjoy a joke—some of them had asked an Irishman whether he knew what "strategy" meant? and he said "Yes, it means like this, sure, when you've fired your last cartridge, don't let the enemy know, but jest kape on firing all the same!" I don't know whether it was original, but he brought it out as though it was.

I have had a few days of slight fever since I wrote last, and I took a couple of days off, and spent them at Umkomaas with some friends, who have a nice cottage down there. It is the most perfect little seaside place I have ever struck; such jolly woods all round the cottage, with semi-tropical growth, and lots of monkeys in the trees; glorious rocks, and *such* a blue sea. I had a delightful rest, and came back much better, but of course found various muddles to face, and they always make one wish one had never gone!

The worst thing I had to straighten out was a complaint from a medical officer about a sister; they had been rubbing each other the wrong way for some time, and of course I thought if I had not gone away I might have kept the peace; however, as the complaint was a definite one (though in no way serious), and was also *just*, I had to move her to a less important ward. This very much hurt her feelings, and I was sorry, as, though not a good manager, she is very good to the patients. Now she works for a different doctor, and there is peace in the camp.

All the civil surgeons and sisters growl at the new military rules and regulations, but I think they are rather inclined to make mountains out of mole-hills—they can really get all they want if they set about it in the proper way, but they don't take the trouble to find out what *is* the proper way. Perhaps I have rather spoilt the sisters by letting them have things that were urgently ordered from my stores at any time, but now that the place is not so crowded up with bad cases they must learn to order in the proper way and at the proper time.

In one respect I was afraid that our system would be changed, but the Major has very kindly arranged it as I wished; I saw, when at the Cape (and heard of it in other hospitals), that when a sick convoy arrived there was much delay before the men were classified and put to bed—sometimes not until several hours after their arrival. One cause of the delay was that each man, if he could crawl, had to go up to the store to draw his kit and sign for it himself; the poor chaps used to look so frightfully ill and tired with this weary waiting about, before they could get food or a wash, after (perhaps) some days in a train.

Here we have managed quite differently; as soon as we received the wire saying that patients were coming (and the number), we had everything issued for that number; the beds were all made up, and before they arrived I used to go round and see that the crockery for each man was on his locker, a clean shirt, towel, soap and flannel, &c., all ready, so that the men could be carried straight to their beds as soon as they arrived, and have a good basin of bovril without any delay; then those who were well enough to go up to the store to give in their kit and to receive their hospital suit did so; and the orderlies took up the kit of those who were too ill (of course they did not want hospital suits).

Now it is necessary for all, who are able, to sign for their equipment (sheets, blankets, &c.); but the Major lets us have some beds fully equipped in each ward before the men arrive, and the orderlies sign for those fittings until the men arrive, and then they countersign the book, so that the bad cases can still be carried straight to their beds.

Our new mess arrangements are working well; it is much more comfortable having a cook with a kitchen separate from that from which all the food for patients, orderlies, and others is served. We had to buy a new stove, but as the expense was shared between the medical officers and sisters, it did not come to very much. Our Madrassee cook is serving us very well. I thought it would be difficult to keep our stores separate, but he seems to manage well and economically, and he is a good cook and serves the things up very nicely. We share the expense of his wages with the doctors, but have separate boys for our mess waiters and for our rooms.

I have kept John on for the sisters' rooms: he is very slow, but a good old thing, and very clean. It is the custom for these boys to go home for a day or two when their wages are paid, but you always keep some of what is due to them in hand (or they don't come back); but when the hospital was handed over to the Government, the boys were all paid up to date, so of course they all cleared, but John promised to come back in two days, and I thought he would; but it was six days later when I found him slinking about his work and looking like a big dog that expected a whipping. I said, "Oh, John, you bad boy, sisters not have you back any more," and then he said his wife was "plenty sick," but I told him I thought Kaffir beer was plenty good, at which he grinned, and I had to forgive him!

William, our good scamp of a mess-room boy, never returned, so I had to go into Durban to the toct (or tax) master at the police station, who generally looks after all the natives and gives them their passes, &c. I chose a boy who was recommended, but he never turned up, so I was thinking I must go again and lead one out from Durban with me, when the dearest little Kaffir turned up, with a note from the toct master, saying he was a very good boy, and his name was "Imdenbe, son of Cholem, Chief of Imsugelum, Umtenta," so I was rather relieved when the boy said his name was "Dick"!

I thought he was much too small to reach to put the things on the table, but he is very quick and nimble and clean, and both the cook and John are very fond of him; so we manage all right, and he looks perfectly sweet in his white suits with red braid—they all wear things like bathing-dresses, with short sleeves, and go about barefoot.

The worst of the enteric season seems to be over now, and we are very slack, and we hear it is the same at all the hospitals up this side. The days are still very hot, but the nights are quite cold.

I expect you hear more about this Hospital Commission than we do, but the R.A.M.C. men are very sick about it, as they have worked so tremendously hard all through the war.

I think every one agrees that the Tommies have never been so well looked after in any war before, but no doubt at the front they have suffered badly, more especially at Bloemfontein, where, suddenly, the army was attacked by a perfect scourge of enteric (I believe there were about 6000 cases there); but people must remember they were 900 miles from their base, with only a single line of rail, and for the last 250 miles almost every bridge destroyed, so that all traffic had to be carried on with the utmost caution over temporary bridges, only a few trucks crossing at a time; also it was an unusually dry season, so that engines often had to drop their heavy trains, run on to get water, and then return for them.

The Transvaal could practically supply nothing to feed the troops, as the Boers had planted no crops.

To get sufficient rations up daily for the men and horses was just about all the one rail could do, and when it was necessary to leave the railway line, the troops often had to wait weeks to scrape together rations to carry with them.

I believe the R.A.M.C. were well prepared for the probable number of wounded, but when unexpected sickness knocked the men over by the thousand, it is scarcely surprising that it was impossible to get up tents and all medical necessaries and comforts quickly enough.

I believe the sick and wounded are quite comfortable now in Bloemfontein; but no doubt there was suffering there, and the Commission will find out whether it might have been prevented.

There can have been little excuse for the bad management that is complained of at the base, and if that is proved, no doubt some one will get blamed for it.

I know the single-line railway on this side, that passes close to us, has been very hard worked night and day; at one time eight trains went up each day with water-tanks only, besides almost incessant trainloads of men, horses, mules, stores, &c.; the only wonder is that there have been so few accidents.

All the sisters have now had some leave, and as we have extra sisters here and very few bad cases, I am going to take a run up-country with a lady from here, and hope to tell you about that next time I write.

XXXIV

I must first of all tell you of my interesting few days up-country. I left here on the evening of the 20th of last month with Mrs. D. and her baby and a small Kaffir nursemaid; she was going to stay with friends who have a hotel and store at Colenso, and I had engaged a bed at this hotel, and took my saddle with me hoping to secure a horse there, and be able to explore the country around.

Two of our medical officers were going for a run up-country the same day, but as the train ran in two sections, I only saw them on the platform at Maritzburg late that evening.

At the same time I saw another officer in khaki looking at me, and then recognised in him a well-known London surgeon who is chief of another hospital out here—of course I was more used to seeing him in frockcoat and top-hat. He had his wife on the train, and as they also were going to Colenso, I was very glad to be able to be with them there.

The train rocked about so much (first crawling up a hill, and then tearing down the other side) that it was difficult to sleep, but the baby slept like an angel with the little Kaffir girl, safely deposited on the floor.

At 4.30 the next morning we arrived at Colenso. It was very cold and very dark, but Mr. Edwards (the hotel proprietor) met us, and with him we stumbled across the veldt to his hotel, which is just a one-storey shanty, as their house had been knocked to pieces by the Boers. Unfortunately he could not possibly take in my friends, so they had to stay at the station.

I was very glad to be able to tumble into a clean bed and have a good sleep, and by breakfast-time I was quite fresh again.

Then I was annoyed to find that I could not get a horse, as they were all engaged, and I had hoped to be able to ride to Ladysmith and to Spion Kop;

however, I got on all right in the end.

That morning we climbed Hlangwane Hill, and saw some really wonderful Boer trenches; you absolutely can see no sign of them in broad daylight till you nearly walk into them.

Then we saw the place where Colonel Long lost his guns (the dead cavalry horses are still lying there); and where poor young Lieutenant Roberts was mortally wounded in trying to save them; and where Major Baptie, R.A.M.C., won his V.C.—I think by carrying Lieutenant Roberts into a donga and staying with him, and other wounded, all through that day of heavy firing, trying to keep them comfortable with some morphia he had with him.

We picked up as many pieces of shells and shrapnel as we could carry, and walked back along the banks of the Tugela.

I heard that a luggage train would be passing at 2.30 P.M., so I thought I would go into Ladysmith by that, and see whether there was any chance of getting out to Spion Kop from there. There are very few passenger trains now (except just the mails), so we are allowed to travel in any train that happens to stop, but of course they don't undertake to keep to any particular time.

Directly after lunch I strolled down to the station—no station-master or any official there, but I met a gentleman who told me that he had walked all the way out from Ladysmith, and was expecting to have to wait for the mail train to take him back, so he was very glad when I told him I knew the next goods train was going to stop there; he said his wife was in the waiting-room, so we walked along to find her, and soon I discovered she was Mrs. ——, Secretary of the Women's Patriotic League in Durban, whom I had not actually met before, but with whom I had had much pleasant correspondence, as they had been very kind in helping us.

So we trained in to Ladysmith together, and on the way they pointed out to me the remains of the great dam which the Boers made to try to flood Ladysmith out, also the neutral camp of Intombi; there is no hospital there now, only the cemetery, sadly full of graves.

They told me they were staying at the "Royal," and that people from there frequently drove out to Spion Kop; so I walked up with them and interviewed the manageress, who told me that a party of ladies had engaged a waggonette to drive out there next morning, and she thought I could easily secure a seat. Eventually I met these ladies, and found they were Durban people who had been over here to help at a concert for our men, so they were very kind and said I had better stay the night (as they had to start early in the morning) and dine with them.

I went out and wired to Colenso not to expect me back, bought a few necessaries, and then took a look round the town.

The hotel I was staying in had had a big shell right through, which had killed a man who was sitting in the hall, and the Town Hall had had a great piece knocked off the tower by one of Long Tom's shells.

Then I climbed up to the convent, which was used at first as officers' quarters, but had been tremendously knocked about by shells. The kind old sisters were very busy with workmen, patching up holes in the walls, &c.

Then I walked out to the cemetery, rather a long walk, and it was getting dusk, so I could not stay long; there were rows and rows of siege graves, and amongst many interesting names I saw those of the Earl of Ava and poor George Stevens of the *Daily Mail*.

It was quite dark when I got back to the hotel, and I was glad of dinner, and not sorry to go early to bed. It is eighteen miles out to Spion Kop, and they won't send a carriage there for less than £5, but for that sum you have four horses, and six people can go in the carriage; I had told the manageress that I would gladly pay £1 for a seat, but in the end I was not allowed to pay anything, as there were only four besides myself, and they had already arranged to pay the £5, and would not let me share.

We started at 6 A.M. with a black driver, and a small white boy to act as guide. Many of the horses that went through the siege have not yet recovered; one of ours was taken worse on the way, and we had to wait while the driver crushed up a nut between two stones and thrust it down the horse's throat, then it struggled on till we reached the kraal at the foot of the hill at 9 A.M., and outspanned. On the way we passed the place where Colonel Dick-Cunyngham was killed.

We had a bite of lunch, and then started with our small guide up the Thaba Inyama, one peak of which is "Spion Kop."

We had with us a January number of the *Natal Mercury* giving a full account of *the* day, so we were able to trace the positions, and I had heard the men talk so much about it I felt I knew my way quite well.

Of course we went up from the Ladysmith side (where the Boers were), but from the top we could look over to Potgieter's Drift and Spearman's Camp, and marvel how our poor chaps ever got up in the dark, with the Boers in such good cover above them; and *then* to be ordered back must have been frightfully disappointing.

We saw many English and Boer graves, and I took a good many photos, including one of the cross on the spot where General Woodgate fell.

We picked up heaps of cartridges (full and empty ones), emergency ration tins, soldiers' uniform buttons, &c.; it was too hard climbing to burden ourselves with any shells, but I bought a few from Kaffirs who had gathered near our carriage. I am collecting a very varied stock of ammunition, including one soft-nosed cartridge.

They were burning the grass down all round the base of the hill, and every now and then a cartridge went off; we hoped the fire would not come across any stray shells while we were there.

We had a splendid view of the Drakensberg Range. Returning to our carriage we had lunch, with an admiring crowd of rather naked Kaffirs around (who seemed much to appreciate our remains), and we started for the return drive about 1 P.M. The sick horse was worse on the way back, and had to have several doses administered.

As we were nearing Ladysmith, I found we were passing close to Tin Town Hospital; so, thinking it was a pity to miss seeing the place, I left the carriage and walked across a drift on the Klip River.

First I passed some officers on their ponies playing at "Heads and Posts"; then I came to the horses' sick camp, and met a nice old veterinary sergeant (who, I found, was a Colonial who came from Kimberley, and of course knew people whom I had met there); he told me he had charge of 400 sick horses, but many of them were "convalescent," and if he had known I wanted a horse he would gladly have lent me one; he said if I would stay another day or two I could send down for my saddle and he would lend me a horse and a mounted orderly so that I could ride to Bulwana, Waggon Hill, Cæsar's Camp, and other places which I should much have liked to visit, but I could not spare the time.

Then he took me along to the sisters' huts. I found the Lady Superintendent was out, but some kindly Kilburn Sisters gave me some tea and took me round the hospital; not many cases in just now, but a few very bad enterics.

The sisters told me that as the Red Cross Ambulance (drawn by eight mules) was going into Ladysmith, I could drive back in it. I was just going to climb inside when a gentleman in khaki came and asked me if I would not rather ride on the top with him, so I gladly climbed up, and found he was a doctor (one of the big civilian doctors); he had heard who I was, and amused me by saying he wished I had called at their mess (fancy shy *me* calling at an unknown officers' mess!) instead of going to tea with "those estimable females," as they would have shown me more of the place, and they have a good collection of curios that would have interested me (he was looking at the things I had picked up). It was a very jolly drive, and he insisted on driving me right up to my hotel.

I must really tell you about the rest of my travels in my next letter. I was away only five days, but you will see that I squeezed a good deal into those days.

XXXV

I will just finish telling you of my travels while they are fresh in my memory, and then this letter can wait till there is enough material to fill it up.

I was very sorry to hear from my friend on the ambulance of the death of Sir William Stokes (physician); he was ill only four days, and it seems only the other day he came round this hospital and was so cheery and bright, and I know he was meaning to say a good deal to the Hospital Commission in favour of the hospitals out here, and of the work they have done.

I just had dinner with my friends at the Royal, and then the 'bus took me to the station with my heavy bag of shells, &c., in time for the 7.40 P.M. train back to Colenso. I was awfully tired, but the mosquitoes were bad, and did not let me have much sleep.

The next day I was invited to go with a picnic party to the Tugela Falls. A large ox waggon was loaded up with children, provisions, &c., and I went with some more people in an Army Service Corps Scotch cart, with no springs, drawn by four mules, who frequently ran away, and who seemed to have a rooted objection to keeping to the road (or rather track); so the journey was rather perilous and distinctly painful.

We passed Fort Wylie, and saw where all the fighting took place on Pieter's Hill, and we saw the rough bridge that the Boers had made over the Tugela by simply pulling up our rails with the sleepers attached and throwing them into the river.

We had lunch close by the Falls—even after this very dry season it is quite a big fall—and after lunch we climbed the hills around, including Hart's Hill. On the top of this hill is a big memorial stone to Colonel Thackery, several more officers, and *sixty-seven* men of the 27th Inniskillings, who fell up there, and we also saw their grave (fenced in) at the foot of the hill.

By the time that we got down to the line again it was blowing a gale, and *such* dust, so some of us sheltered in a platelayer's cottage.

He had a fine collection of shells and other relics; his cottage had been used by the Boers as a telegraph station, and we found he had been in the smash-up of the armoured train, when Winston Churchill was taken prisoner.

As Mrs. D. had her baby with her, and it was now a really bad dust-storm, this man kindly stopped a goods train with his red flag, and we returned comfortably to Colenso in the guard's van.

I should much like to have had longer stay both at Colenso and Ladysmith, there was so much of interest both in the places and in the people one met; but I wanted to visit a few places on the way down, so I left Colenso the next morning at 9.30. My first stop was at Chieveley, where there had been a big hospital, but all that remains now is a little closed-in graveyard, with nearly two hundred graves; many died from wounds, but many more from enteric. They had a clever way of marking the graves, each man's name, regiment, &c., being written on a slip of paper and enclosed in a medicine bottle and securely stuck into the mound.

I saw poor Lieutenant Roberts' grave (it has a plain stone with an inscription, but I hear a cross is being sent out); they had brought him from Colenso on the ambulance train the evening of the day he was wounded. The station-master told me he had helped to lift him out of the train, and he seemed sensible and comfortable then, but he died the same night.

I saw a very fine redoubt at Chieveley made by the Royal Engineers, but it was never used. I took the next train on to Mooi River. Before we reached Frere station we passed the place of the armoured train disaster, and the graves of the Royal Dublin Fusiliers who fell there. Wherever you go there seem to be graves dotted about, most of them enclosed with barbed wire, and some with a cross set up, or the man's initials marked out in empty cartridge-cases.

There is a large hospital at Estcourt, but I had only time for a hasty lunch at the station there, as I wanted to have an hour or two at Mooi River, to see the hospital, where I knew one of the doctors, and where it seemed probable that we should be sent when we first arrived; on the whole, I am glad we were *not* stationed there, though they have had more interesting surgical work than we have.

Unfortunately my friend was away, but the superintendent kindly showed me round, and I had tea in the sisters' mess.

They have 950 beds, nearly all under canvas. It was blowing hard, and while I was there it began to rain, and it was snowing on the Drakensberg, and very cold, so every one looked rather miserable. It is a desolate place on the bare veldt.

I left again on a goods train at 4.30, and rattled down to Maritzburg by 9 P.M., where I meant to stay the night.

Miss —— kindly met me at the station, and we drove down to her house in a riksha; she has been taking in convalescent nurses, and feeding them and giving them a rest. She has had much anxiety about her brothers, one of whom was commandeered and had to fight for the Boers, together with his son (a boy of sixteen). They were with Cronje at Paardeberg, and are now prisoners at St. Helena; another brother was fighting for us, and was taken prisoner by the Boers, but released when we took Pretoria.

Miss —— wanted me to go out to Howick to see the falls there, and to have a look at the big convalescent camp, where they have 1600 beds; but the train left half-an-hour earlier than she thought, so I missed it, and instead she took me to see the Maritzburg Hospitals, Fort Napier, Grey's Hospital (now civilian again), and the Garrison Church, the last the most comfortable looking hospital I have seen further up-country than this one, but it was a little strange to see the men in their hospital suits lounging and smoking on the church steps.

I met a sister whom I had known in London. She was excited about playing in a cricket match; and as she and all the eleven sisters had been given a week's leave from duty to practise for this cricket match, they are evidently as slack in the way of work as we are.

I had some nice greetings from some old patients of ours, now on duty in Maritzburg.

I left there about 6 P.M., had dinner at Inchanga with a *Daily News* correspondent, and got back here about 9.30 P.M. Some orderlies were at the station and kindly carried up my load of curios, &c.

The two medical officers had got back the night before, and though they went as far up as Newcastle they had not seen as much as I had, and regretted that they had not had my offer of a convalescent horse at Ladysmith!

I have seen a good many hospitals, and met a good many sisters, and I have gathered a few hints of little ways in which we might improve this hospital; but, though "I says it as shouldn't," I don't think there is any hospital up this side where the men are more comfortable and happy, and I think the sisters here are better fed and their mess bills are no higher than at any of the hospitals—indeed, lower than most of them.

I was glad to find that they had had a peaceful time while I was away, and no difficulties; and as there are actually only eighteen men and ten officers in, we are still very slack; we expect some more any day now, but there is very little sickness just at present.

You ask about the men and their letters; it was rather difficult when we were so frightfully busy at first to do all that one would have liked, but we always try to write for the men who are too ill to write for themselves, and I always saw that all the men who wished had writing materials, and they used to help each other.

They say at some of the base hospitals stray lady visitors have been such a nuisance in interfering with the nurses, but I could well and safely have employed a few stray ladies in amusing the men, writing their letters for them, &c. The friends of those officers who were dangerously ill were all written to by each mail.

Now that we are slack, of course, I have much more chance of talking to the men, and they tell me many tales of the fighting, and of the rough time they have had at the front; but you will hear plenty of that from the men who have gone home.

I am beginning to have many grateful letters from our patients' friends at home.

There has been some delay about our pay lately, and some of the sisters who were lodging here had not received any since they left England, so were not able to pay their mess bills, and I had to pay various mess accounts when I got back from my run up-country, and began to feel rather anxious as to whether I could go on feeding my large party of sisters; but now the pay has turned up, so we have got straight again; and the Government give us various allowances—Colonial allowance, and for mess, servants, fuel, &c., so we are feeling rather well off.

We are much enjoying a big package of papers that the Red Cross Society now send up to us each week; whole weeks of *Times*, *Daily Mail*, *Daily Graphic*, *Daily Telegraph*, *Standard*, *Illustrated London News*, *Army and Navy*, &c. They are the greatest boon to the whole camp.

The men point out to me the "pretty boys" in the illustrated papers when they see any pictures of soldiers, as, by comparison, they all look so thin and rough out here.

XXXVI

Now we are really getting busy again. Patients keep arriving, sometimes small parties, sometimes large.

Early in September we admitted thirteen men who had been prisoners in Pretoria for nine months. They were very weak and run down, and so happy to be here; when I took them their first basket of fruit, they simply wolfed it down, as they had seen no fruit since they went up-country.

Then we had rather a "difficult" batch of officers sent down from Mooi River. They have no officers' wards there, so these men had been quartered in a hotel more than a mile from the hospital, where each had his own room and servant, and they seem to have ordered and done just what they liked.

Up to now we have never had more than three or four officers well enough to sit up to meals at one time, as they have always come to us really ill, and as soon as they were well enough they have either rushed back to the front or have been sent home on the hospital ships; but with these officers from Mooi River (none of them very ill), I suddenly found that we had twenty-four sick officers in, and that *sixteen* of them were well enough to sit up to meals, and that it was not suitable for them to eat in the ward where there were a few men still very ill; so, eventually, a large tent had to be rigged up for them, and as it was a long way from the kitchen there was some difficulty in getting the food to them hot.

The medical officer was a civilian, and he did not seem to think he had anything to do with the responsibility about feeding these hungry convalescent officers; in fact, every one seemed rather inclined to say "It isn't my work"—and our St. John's men are not like R.A.M.C. men, who may be accustomed to turning to as mess waiters on occasion; neither was the cook quite ready to serve up a dinner of several courses instead of single "diets" for each patient.

I am afraid I had to worry the poor C.O.; but I knew if I did not do so the officers would complain they could not get anything to eat; and, after wrestling through the first night's dinner—(when I found well-meaning orderlies running down with the fish before the soup, and some vegetables after the sweets had been served!)—we laid plans for better management, and for a day or two the Major went to the kitchen and saw the food sent down in proper order, and I received it and saw it served in the tent, and four of the officers' servants were told off to wait each night, and the orderlies had only to carry the food down for them. So now that is running all right, and I only just have to look in to see they have all they want.

For some time we have been expecting to be inspected by the Hospital Commission, but at last we heard they were not coming here at all, as there had been "no complaints" about this hospital; so I should have been very vexed if our record had been spoilt at this late stage of the war.

Our next order was to prepare for a train that was bringing us seven officers and 108 men from Pretoria (the biggest trainload we have yet received). Having had sisters here over our correct number for some time, and very little for them to do, of course as soon as we got busy we kept having wires to send one sister for duty on the Hospital Ship *Avoca*, or two sisters to the Hospital Ship *Dunera*, and so on, and none of them wanted to go, so it was a little difficult to sort them.

In fact, there have been so many orders and counter orders that I should never be surprised if I had a wire telling me to go off on a hospital ship, or if we had orders to pack up the whole hospital and take it up to Pretoria.

Before Mr. X. left, he let us buy some remaining groceries at home prices (a great saving for our mess), and after we found a small storeroom to arrange them in, I, rather foolishly, let them use the cases for firewood, which has been very scarce here; so, if we have to move, all the sisters intend to sling bottles of fruit, and tins of jam, sardines, &c., round them, as we really can't leave our stores behind!

I hear that the army sisters on the hospital ships are rather horrified that I am still left in charge here, now that it is a Military Hospital, and that there are plenty of army sisters out in the country; but the P.M.O. has been very nice to me, and I am very glad to "carry on" as long as they want me; the only thing is that I should very much have liked to see a little of the work nearer up to the front, and as it seems probable that this place will become, later on, a sort of convalescent home, the work will not be so interesting.

Yesterday some officers went down to Durban, and came back much excited by rumours that the line and the wire had been cut at Standerton, that 1700 Boer prisoners had been released, that Johannesburg was surrounded, and a few more exciting items, but I dare say they are not true; I never pretend to tell you about the war.

By degrees we are getting a few R.A.M.C. orderlies and non-commissioned officers, and of course they make the work easier for us; but we are quite proud of some of the St. John's men, who are becoming excellent and most efficient nurses, and they really knew nothing of nursing six months ago.

I had a great triumph when the big batch of men (108) arrived, as everything had been issued for them the day before and signed for by the orderlies, and half-an-hour after they arrived every man was either comfortably in bed or had had a preliminary wash and was ready to sit down to a good meal, and after that he went up to the store to hand in his kit; some of the patients and some of the R.A.M.C. men told me that in many of the Military Hospitals it would have taken four or five hours to get so many of them settled and fed.

There are several very bad cases amongst them, but also a good many convalescents. We have two officers desperately ill, one a Major in the R.A.M.C., who, I fear, is not likely to get better, though they are trying everything possible for him, and the other is a Lieutenant in the Rifle Brigade who has been delirious for a long time (enteric) and very ill, but I fancy he will pull round. I have been able to give him special nurses when necessary. Also we have a bad case of enteric in the men's ward; I don't think I have ever seen a case where there has been so much hæmorrhage, and yet I think he will pull round, though he is nearly a skeleton, and even I can easily lift him up while his sheet is changed. I have been much pleased at the really tender way the orderlies have nursed this boy, as he has needed a great deal of patience.

We are getting quite keen on our gardens now that we have a little more time to breathe, but whenever I plant anything I wonder whether, by any chance, I shall be here to see it grow up. I now have some healthy violets and some ivy-leaf geraniums. Some time ago I had two beautiful Orpington hens and a cock given to me. They lay splendidly, and the eggs have been very useful, but they showed no sign of wishing to sit, so I got a friend to put some of my eggs under a broody hen, and hope soon to have some young Orpingtons.

The men have not had time to make me a henhouse yet, so we have to keep a sharp look-out to secure the eggs, and our small Dick is very attentive to them.

I went into Durban the other day to do some shopping for the mess, and saw some friends, and then I went down to the jetty to see some of our orderlies and patients (a nice lot of men of the Coldstreams and other regiments, many of them wounded from Pretoria), who were going home on the *Montrose*. I met a sister whom I knew, and one of our medical officers was seeing the men on board, and one of the embarkation people invited us to go out in the tender to the *Montrose* at the outer anchorage; so we had a nice little sea breeze, and the officers on board gave us tea, and offered to show us our cabins, so we had a good chance to stow away for home!

Six of our orderlies were going home on duty, and they all came to say good-bye, and we had quite a "send off" from them and the old patients when we left the ship.

To-day some people have been giving a picnic at a pretty place called Krantz Kloof. They invited all we could spare to join them, so I let six sisters go, and four of the medical officers and four convalescent officers also went off with them in an ox waggon at 8 A.M., and they did not get back till 9 P.M. I have been busy all day keeping an eye on the place generally to see that nothing was neglected while so many were away.

The night sister and night special both went, so I have now sent them to bed for a few hours, and I have been writing beside Lieutenant —— (of the Rifle Brigade), but I am sure he is better to-day, and to-night he is inclined to sleep; every now and then I let the orderly sit by him while I take a prowl round to see the other wards are all right; now it is 2 A.M., so I shall call the two sisters and turn in, and I need not hurry up in the morning unless there are any fresh orders to attend to.

XXXVII

PINETOWN, NATAL,
October 1900.

We have had a good deal of rain lately and the country is looking lovely again: you can almost see the things growing in the garden.

Sometimes it rains for three days without stopping, and South Africa without the sun always looks very gloomy, but when the sun comes out again it makes up for the gloominess.

It has begun to get very hot rather earlier than usual, and the thermometer showed 94° in the shade the other day.

Last month we took in fifty more men who had been prisoners with the Boers; a good many of them were gentlemen troopers of the Yeomanry; they were sent here *via* Delagoa Bay; one of them brought a parrot, and there were several small birds as well.

Then the other day we took in eighty men from Charlestown, nearly all convalescents, and such a mixed lot of regiments—Scotch, Irish, Australians, New Zealanders, and Tasmanians, and one little Australian bugler, aged fifteen, whom all the men spoil.

The poor Major of the R.A.M.C., who I told you was so ill, died in the early part of this month; it was very sad, as he knew so well what all the bad symptoms meant as they appeared.

I think I told you also of Lieutenant ——, who was desperately ill for so long. We had a very anxious time with him, as the delirium went on for so long that we began to fear it would become permanent, but at last he pulled round, and has been such a nice patient. We have very few officers in now.

The Natal Volunteers were expected to return to Durban on October 2nd (they have been a year at the front), but the Boers attacked a convoy near Dundee, and they were all ordered back.

Durban was preparing a great welcome for them, and the meat for the big lunch that the Mayor was going to give them was actually cooked! They got home about a week later, and we all went down to the station to see them pass, many of our old patients amongst them.

I had the bad luck to have a nasty fall out riding early in the month, and am only beginning to crawl about again, with a good deal of pain from a damaged kidney. One of the medical officers was ill, and had asked me to exercise his pony any time I liked to use it (he didn't like the Kaffir boy taking it out), so, when the Major and another man asked me to go with them to pay a few calls on people who have been very kind to us here, I thought it would be a good chance to exercise the pony. From here down to the station is a good bit of soft sand, and all the ponies were fresh, so we let them scatter along; then I saw there was a train shunting at the level crossing, so I wanted to pull up before we got mixed up on the line (of course no gates here), and just then one of the men lost his hat; my pony got cross at being checked, and bucked a bit, and then suddenly swung round and jumped a fallen tree, and off I went on the wrong side, falling across a branch of the tree. I can't think why I fell, except that I was so sure I could not come off, I never thought about sticking on, and was preparing to give him a licking for being so stupid.

I did not feel much damaged at the time, though I thought I should have a big bruise just above my hip, and when they had caught my pony I remounted and we went on again; luckily most of the people were out, but at one place I had to get off, and when it came to remounting I simply could not spring, and had to condescend to mount from a chair, and when I got home I felt really bad and had to go to bed.

Fortunately there were plenty of sisters to do the work, and things went on all right while I was laid up, and now I can get about enough to do the housekeeping, and hope soon to get round the wards again, but they are very quiet at present.

We have rather amusing "tiffs" between the officers' and sisters' mess; just now potatoes are very scarce, as the military people have bought them all up; I found the cook was using mine for the officers, as they had run out, so I told them I had had to pay 32s. 6d. for a bag, but I should charge them more by the pound! they thought I had paid too much, and asked the C.O., who was going into Durban to bring them out a bag. When he came back, he had to confess that he had had to give 35s. for a bag, and it never turned up at the station, and he had no receipt, and did not know the name of the shop!

We are constantly having to make little exchanges of food, &c., but it is necessary to keep a very sharp eye on our supplies.

Our nice little imp, Dick—otherwise Imdenbe, son of Cholem, Chief of Imsugelum, Umtenta—got home-sick, and wanted to go home to his mother, so now we have another boy for the mess-room. I dare say Dick will come slinking back when he has spent his money.

John, the big house-boy, is still here, and is an excellent servant. When we first came, Mr. —— let him take care of his horse (of course paying him extra), but then, when other medical officers also got horses, the Major said that one boy must look after them all—as there were difficulties about fodder, &c.—but when Mr. —— told John, he said, "No, sir, me never give up Tommy; Tommy he clean, he fat, he happy, and John love him; John cry very much if boss give Tommy one new boy." But poor John had to give him up; and I believe he *did* cry. In my room I have the luxury of a big wardrobe with glass doors, and John takes great pride in this piece of furniture; I believe he loves to see himself in the mirror. One day I found he had turned my dresses out to dust inside—I expected him to proceed to tidy the drawers next, but I drew the line there! He keeps our rooms beautifully clean, and is absolutely honest. The other day he knocked at one of the sister's doors when she was having a bath, and when she told him he could not come in, he said "It's only me, old John," and was quite hurt that she would not unlock the door.

I think I told you about his going home after payday and stopping too long: the same thing happened again the other day, and when he came slinking round with his broom and pail again (looking as though he expected me to hit him), I said, "Oh, John, I just going to toctmaster for another boy," and he said, "No, missus, me never leave the sisters, but my wife very sick, and it rain very much, and—Kaffir beer very good at my kraal," so I had to forgive him, as he was honest about it!

We have had a good many changes amongst the sisters lately, but at present they seem a happy lot, and they work well; they have been much more contented since they took their few days up-country, as it has made them realise that in most ways they are better off here.

As the summer comes on, the creeping and crawling beasts are getting very objectionable; amongst others that come into my room are grasshoppers, locusts, flying beetles (huge brutes), and mosquitoes. When they get very numerous, I have to turn my light off and wait till I hear them all make for the electric light outside.

There are six cats about the place, and two of them insist on sleeping in my room (of course my door and window are always open); one always sleeps on my chest of drawers, and the other on the clothes basket, so I feel safe that snakes won't come in, as a cat always lets you know when one is about.

One night the small tabby brought the most extraordinary creature into my room: it was like a small crab, and it ran round and round in a circle, and squeaked like one of those clock-work mice.

The other day it began to rain, and then we were afflicted by a perfect scourge of flying ants, which I had never seen before in such numbers.

They covered the walls of our rooms, and some of the sisters could eat no dinner, as they were so thick on the mess-room table. The men in the wards swept them up in bucketfuls; then, in a couple of hours, they all took themselves off again, without any apparent method in their madness.

We have all sorts of vegetables and flowers coming on in the garden, the rainy weather suiting them well, but the wet days are rather dull for the men, and there seems to be more sickness starting again up-country.

I had a letter from J. the other day from Kroonstad, saying that he was fit and well, but heartily sick of trekking about the Free State. Really *all* the men seem so tired of the war just now; it is all very well to put up with hardships, and short rations, for a few months, but when it runs on to a year, every one has had enough.

The other day we had a wire to ask for a doctor to go to an officer who had been taken ill when on leave about an hour up the line from here. Dr. ——

went to see him and found him rather bad, so the next day a stretcher-party went up and brought him here. We have several rather bad cases in just now, but we have plenty of people to look after them, and there is none of the anxiety we had at first, when we were overwhelmed with enteric cases, and the orderlies were so helpless.

We hear that Lord Roberts is coming down this way soon, but there are so many rumours that we hardly know what to believe.

XXXVIII

Of course you will have heard that poor Prince Christian Victor died at Pretoria of enteric. He was buried in the military cemetery there, and there was a service in the cathedral; I heard it was very impressive—about 1000 troops attended.

I should like to have been in Pretoria when the Proclamation declaring the annexation of the Transvaal was read. I heard it was very fine. Lord Roberts arrived with a big escort (including some fine Indians), and massed bands played "God Save the Queen," and then the Royal Standard was run up, and then again "God Save the Queen." After that there were no less than six Victoria Crosses for Lord Roberts to pin on—he stood on the steps of the old Dutch church—and then there was a march past of 10,000 troops. I believe the march past took two hours, though the infantry left the Square at the "double."

It is very difficult to judge, but many people here seem to think the war is by no means over yet; however, if Lord Roberts does go home, we shall have K. of K. to finish the business.

The chief thing of interest here early in the month was some difficulty about the three civil surgeons who were still here (of those who came out with us). There has been some muddle since the Government took over the hospital, as to whether they were to have the pay of medical officers engaged at home or of those engaged out here; after some correspondence they were dissatisfied with the terms, and thought they were being hardly treated; and then a wire came that they were to prepare to proceed to England, as their services were no longer required. I expect they will get the matter settled all right when they get home.

It was quite a business getting them all packed up in a hurry, and they had to arrange about selling their horses, &c.

They gave a farewell dinner-party, which we all attended.

The Army Medical Department is a bit unsettling; of course you have to do exactly what you are told, and you are told to do things so suddenly: just a wire comes, and very often next day you move.

Colonel Galway (the P.M.O.) has gone home, and we miss him very much; he has been so particularly nice every time he has been here.

We have had a very quiet time lately. They are closing some beds up at Maritzburg, and sent us down a very good wardmaster and fifteen R.A.M.C. orderlies—some of them men with six or seven years' service.

At first the sisters could hardly realise that these men were really good nurses, as they have been so used to having to do most of the nursing themselves until they had shown each particular orderly how to do things; so they think now that the army sisters, in time of peace, must have a very easy life!

One night we had some people to dinner, and then they gave the men such a good concert. Some of the orderlies helped—one of them plays the violin beautifully, and the little Australian boy "bugled."

Another day a clergyman, who has a boys' school up the line, brought all his boys down to pay us a visit, and they played a cricket match against the medical officers and orderlies.

One other form of amusement has been very popular with the men, though rather an unusual one for hospital patients; we have a Lieutenant of the R.A.M.C. on duty here now, and when he went to the remount depot to secure a horse, he was rather surprised that a very nice-looking beast was willingly handed over to him when he said he would like it; but when they got it up here it promptly chucked all the stableboys in turn, and proved to be a bad Australian buckjumper!

Then the men, patients and orderlies, wanted to try their hand with him, and some of the Australian Bushmen are splendid at sticking on. Now he is getting quite tame, and only bucks a little when they first mount. The daily riding of the buckjumper has amused the whole camp; and I should simply have loved to try my hand at sticking on, but my damaged side won't allow me to ride anything for some time yet, though I am getting about my work all right, going slow.

They have had a very "mixed" lot of horses out here, and many people seem to think the war might have been over now if they had had a better supply of horses at first.

The English chargers have worked awfully well, but the food of the country has not been suitable for them, and the little Boer ponies are much better suited for the rough ground and the poor food.

They are so used to picking their way on the veldt that they hardly ever put a foot into a hole; and then at night they will peck about and nibble odds and ends at which an English horse turns up his nose.

At first the men did not think the Boer ponies were big enough to carry the necessary weight, but now they find they are, and that they wear better, because they are not always hungry, as seems to be the case with the unfortunate big horses. Still, the good old London 'bus horses have done very useful work with the guns.

They have had many horses from New Zealand, Australia, and the Argentine—these last often very bad-tempered beasts.

As the men all seem so well satisfied with these Boer ponies, it might be a good plan after the war to start a big Government breeding station out here, in some bit of healthy grass country. A man told me they could ship horses to England for about £20 for the voyage, and that if it was undertaken in a proper way, it ought not to cost more than about £5 to rear a horse, or perhaps £7 to put a four-year-old on board ship, so they could have one of the best landed in England for under £30, where there is so much trouble about getting the right kind of horses in sufficient numbers. They would be suitable for work in almost any climate, as they have to put up with such rapid changes of temperature here.

We have lately had a R.A.M.C. Major here, partly as a patient and partly as a visitor. He was in Ladysmith through the siege, and had very hard work (so many doctors ill); then he was sent down to a hospital ship as a patient, and very soon the C.O. was called away, and he was put in charge while still ill. He has been three trips in her, and seems to have had a lot of work and worry, and now he is ordered to go up and take charge of a 500-bed hospital, and is not in the least fit for it. They won't spare any R.A.M.C. men to be invalided home just now, as they seem to want to weed out all the civil surgeons first. This man wants the most careful feeding to get him right; at first I was always running after him with egg flips or some little feed, but now he is beginning to enjoy ordinary food better.

I have heard a good deal about the siege from him: he tells me it was awful being responsible for sick men and not being able to get things for them. At one time he had 400 very sick under his charge, and all he could get for them was five, or sometimes six, small tins of condensed milk a day, when they all needed milk. He says that the men had no time to convalesce: it was three days up and out of bed, and then straight to the trenches; the poor fellows were so awfully weak that they used to have to send a mule waggon to cart them down. They put a rifle in their hands, and carted them back again at night.

For a short time, too, we had another Major for a "rest and feed up"; he is an M.P. when he is at home, but was out here with the Yeomanry. He is also on the mend now.

I have had the very sweetest puppy given to me—a little black spaniel. He has been christened "Bobs," and he follows me about everywhere.

I must tell you a little joke about some officers who were here. There is a big Convalescent Depot at Howick, and no one seems to like going there, but at one time we were so full up with officers (and more wanting to come), that the Major chose out three or four who were practically well, but not quite fit to rough it at the front yet, and sent them up to Howick. We gave them some sandwiches and fruit to console them on the way, and at Maritzburg they bought a bottle of champagne, and were having a great lunch in the train. There was one little man in plain clothes in the carriage besides our party, so they invited him to lunch, but he refused. While they were lunching they were all talking about what a good time they had had here, and what hard luck it was that the C.O. had pitched on them to go up to the "Home for Lost Dogs" (as Howick is called)—every one said it was a horrid hole, and of course they exaggerated all the bad things they had heard about it. When they got to Howick the little man in plain clothes got out, and an orderly came up and saluted and took his bag, and he proved to be the Colonel in charge at Howick!

We sent off sixty men on the 21st, and, a few days later had seventy men down from Standerton, all supposed to be convalescents, but two of them have developed definite enteric, and as they have been at Standerton for some time ill with something else, they must have become infected up there. I am afraid enteric is getting rather bad again farther up, but of course there always is more at this season, and they are better prepared to tackle it now.

The big hospital at Estcourt has been moved up to Pretoria, and I believe the beds at Maritzburg have been reduced from 1600 to 200; and now we hear that they are having rather a scare lest they should be short of beds on this side.

The other day a man from the Ordnance Department came up to see about putting new sinks in the theatre and otherwise improving the buildings, so that does not look as though we were to close just yet; but I think if the place is kept going into the New Year they are bound to send an Army Superintendent in my place, as it would be too "irregular" to leave me here now that there are so many army sisters about (with some hospitals already closed), and not by any means all of them acting as superintendents.

XXXIX

We have had an exciting time since I last wrote to you; I had better begin at the beginning, and tell you of the upheaval.

At the beginning of the month we heard that the P.M.O. was hovering near, so we thought he would come to inspect us, and then we should learn our fate.

Instead of that, one Sunday our Major had a wire asking him to go down to see the P.M.O. in Durban the next morning "on urgent business." Every one was so excited on Monday they did not know how to work, and I saw that all the medical officers were ready to waylay the poor Major as soon as he got back, so I kept out of the way, thinking he would be tired, and that we should hear the news after he had had some tea.

But very soon he came to my room and said, "Well, Sister, would you like to go to England to-morrow?" I only *said*, "No, sir, not particularly; I think it would be rather cold there just now, and I should like to see the war through," but I *thought* to myself, "What has gone wrong that he wants to ship me off?" because we had worried through some very thick times of difficulties together; but then he explained to me that *he* had been chosen to go home in charge of the sick on the ship on which Lord Roberts was to go —the *Canada*—and he was to choose two sisters and some good orderlies to take with him; he thought the trip would do me good, as I had not been really well since my accident, and he thought I could certainly come out again if I wished, but (of course) I should very likely not get back here as Superintendent. I did not mind that at all, as for some time I had been keen on seeing some work farther up-country, and it seems likely that this place will become more of a "Rest Camp," and less of an acute hospital as time goes on.

Anyhow, he seemed to wish me to go with him, so in ten minutes I had made up my mind to go, and we had decided to take Sister —— (one of our original batch of sisters) with us; and then there were the orderlies to choose.

It was 5.30 P.M. on Monday when I got my marching orders, and the Major had to leave the next day at 12.17, and we to follow him at 3.40 P.M., so you can imagine we had a rush, and there was little sleep for us that night.

The R.A.M.C. Lieutenant was put in temporary charge until the P.M.O. could send a Major down; my senior sister took over the Superintendent's duty for me, and I had to show her all the details about the mess accounts, stores, linen, washing, &c.; arrange to send my dog back to the people who had given him to me (as I should not have been able to land him in England); send my saddle up to Maritzburg to be sold, so as to make room in my saddle-box for packing curios, &c.; to say nothing of my own packing up, and heaps of other things to arrange about.

I could not go to see any of the many friends who had been so kind to us; but before the ship sailed I was able to write fifteen letters of farewell and apologies, and managed to send them ashore.

There was a good deal to settle about the servants too: our good Madrassee cook was to leave the next day, and all the black boys said they "no stay if the big boss and the little missus go to England"; but perhaps they will settle down again.

All the orderlies came crowding down to the station to see us off, and gave us such cheers; and John and the other black boys were all mopping their eyes, Charlie holding on to my little Bobs, who was whining and struggling to come with me—but he will go back to a very good home.

When we got on board at Durban we found the ship had to go to the outer anchorage. We were disappointed that we could not even go up the town to say good-byes, and really we might have had another night ashore, as Lord Roberts never came down till the next day.

Our good friend, Mr. T., from Pinetown, kindly came on board to say good-bye, and brought us a lovely hamper of flowers, some of which we arranged in Lord Roberts' cabin.

Fifty men were to leave the day after we did, so they will be very light in the hospital, and the P.M.O. said he should not send more down till he had settled the staff.

Lord Roberts came on board with his staff at 6 P.M. on December 5th, and we sailed at once. Only 400 troops came on board at Durban, but we heard we should have 1200 after Cape Town.

The *Canada* is a splendid boat, with the finest stretch of upper deck that I have seen on any ship. From Durban to Cape Town the saloon was very empty; besides Sister and myself there was only one lady on board, the wife of a chaplain from Wynberg—they have been to Ceylon for a trip with a shipload of Boer prisoners.

Besides Lord Roberts, we have on board General Ian Hamilton, General Kelly-Kenny, General Marshall, Lord Stanley, and others.

I was shown a copy of the orders about the Medical Company to be put on board this ship: it read, "to include two specially selected sisters"—it sounded like choosing turkeys for Christmas!

There is a hospital with eighty-four cots on board, but, as the men were supposed to be chiefly time-expired men and not sick troops, we did not expect very much work.

We had fine weather coming round the coast, and Lord Roberts went ashore to receive addresses both at East London and at Port Elizabeth; after Port Elizabeth there was a very heavy swell till we reached Cape Town, and poor Sister —— was so bad we were quite glad the hospital was still empty.

Before we reached Cape Town Lord Roberts came up to speak to me, and we had quite a long chat; he was very anxious that we should have everything that we wanted for the hospital.

He told me that Lady Roberts and his two daughters would join us at Cape Town; and two sisters who have been nursing her are coming home with the Miss Roberts who has been ill.

At Cape Town Lord Roberts had a great reception, of which I got some good photos. When I could get away from the ship I went up the town and wired to my brother in Kimberley, to tell him that I was going home, but after doing so I thought I might as well inquire whether, by any chance, he was down in Cape Town, so I went to his club, and was much surprised to find he was in the town; so I left a note to arrange to meet him next day.

The next day was Sunday, and Sister and I went to service in the cathedral (which Lord Roberts attended with his staff), and then my brother met us, and took us up to an excellent lunch at Mount Nelson Hotel.

After lunch Sister —— went off to see some friends at Wynberg, and my brother and I went to see various friends in the suburbs, and finished up with supper with the S.'s at their lovely Kenilworth home. It was nice meeting so many old friends; and then I went back to sleep on board.

The next morning I made a raid on the Red Cross Society and the "Absent Minded Beggar" people to beg for games, cards, books, tobacco, &c., for the men on the way home; and in a few hours' time they sent me on a splendid supply. Then it was "Ladies' Day" at the club, so I found time to run up to lunch with my brother there, and he had some old Kimberley friends also lunching with him. After that the troops were coming on board, so I had to go back to duty.

I was appointed Lady Superintendent for the voyage, and two more sisters were sent on to help us—also three Roman Catholic sisters who had been nursing in Bloemfontein, had a passage home on the *Canada*, and were to be "available for duty" if I wanted them.

The Cape Town people gave Lord Roberts a great send off on December 10th, and H.M.S. *Doris* escorted us out to sea.

We have very comfortable cabins, and the Major (who is P.M.O. on board) invited Sister —— and me to sit at his table in the saloon with four other officers, so we are well looked after.

A great many of the men are wounded, some of them going home for operations. We had twenty sent straight into the hospital before we sailed, and we soon began to fill up there and to get busy.

Before we reached St. Helena one poor fellow of the Yeomanry had died; he did not seem particularly bad when he came on board, but he came down to the hospital saying he felt "a bit queer"; his temperature was only 100°, but we admitted him at once, and he was evidently just beginning a relapse (enteric), and then he had a dreadful septic abscess and other complications, so we had to isolate him in a little cabin, to reach which we had to go past all the stables—there were several horses on board, including the charger poor Lieutenant Roberts was riding when he fell. He was so bad one evening that Sister —— volunteered to sit up with him, but when I went to relieve her at 7 A.M. we could both see that he was dying, and Sister offered to stay so that I should not infect myself; but she looked so done up (she is a bad sailor) I thought she had had enough, and the other sisters could quite well manage the hospital, so I sent her to disinfect, and go to bed.

The poor man died about 10 A.M., and was buried in the afternoon, Lord Roberts and all his staff attending. I don't think anything is more solemn than a funeral at sea; the slow march out to the stern, and the service read, and then the engines stop, and there is such a hush when the constant beat of the screw ceases; next the little splash as the body, heavily weighted and sewn up in a blanket, slides into the sea, and then the mournful "Last Post" sounded: once more the engines start, and we all go back to our posts.

I did not put on a regular night sister except when there was special need; but we took it in turns to be responsible for a night at a time, and the responsible one stayed up till twelve, and then (if all was quiet) turned in, and was called again at 4 A.M. to take a look round; but if she was kept up much, we relieved her from duty for the next morning; we had very good orderlies, and we found this plan worked well.

XL

S.S. "CANADA" (nearing ST. HELENA, on return voyage to the CAPE), *January 1901*.

I am now on my way back to the Cape after sixteen days' leave in England; a rushing time, amid snow and sleet; but I must first tell you about the voyage home.

We reached St. Helena on December 16th, and Lord Roberts and nearly every one went ashore for a few hours. I did not go off as I was busy in the hospital. Several men were very ill with enteric, and one with double pneumonia; of course it was frightfully stuffy for them in the hospital, but Lord Roberts had most kindly said that we were to use part of the upper deck (that had been reserved for him and his family), if it would be any better for the men; so we rigged up a screen, and put two or three men, who seemed most in need of fresh air, up there, and they were so grateful.

There was always a good supply of ice, and the sterilised milk was good; one man (who was very ill) could not take it, but for him I was able to get fresh milk, as there were two cows on board. The "skoff" for the convalescents was excellent, and they were all delighted with the variety of food supplied by the company, after the sameness of the army rations. Both the ship's officers and the stewards were most kind in every way in helping me to get what I wanted for the men.

We had a spell of very hot weather between the 16th and the 21st, and on the 20th we had another sad death, a young St. John's Ambulance man, who was admitted on the 16th with acute rheumatism (he had had enteric in South Africa). It was my night on duty, and at 11.45 I did not think he seemed so well, and I found his temperature had run up to 105°, and his pulse was very bad; we did everything that was possible for the poor boy, but his temperature continued to rise and his heart to fail; he was dreadfully breathless, and it was so difficult to prop him up enough in the bunks; by 1 A.M. his temperature had reached 106.6°, and he knew that he was dying, and was able to tell me where to write to his mother. He died very soon after.

It was dreadfully sad for the other men, as, of course, they were all awake, and in such terribly close quarters—one man in the bunk above him, and two more close beside him; and it does seem such hard luck for these two men to have got through their time in South Africa and then to knock over just when they are nearing home.

A nice sergeant in a bunk near by saw that I was very much cut up about this poor boy, and said, "Never mind, Sister, no one could have done more for the poor lad to give him a chance than you have; but I know I have seen many men die on the battlefield, but it's a lot worse to see one die between decks here." Afterwards we carried him out to a small bathroom, and he was buried the next day.

I found one of the patients in the hospital was a Bart.'s student who had been serving at the front.

Both Lord and Lady Roberts took a great interest in the men, and Lord Roberts used to come up to me in the morning and ask how they had got through the night; and he would ask after the men who were especially ill by name: of course they were awfully pleased when I told them.

They both went round the hospital several times, and on Christmas Day they went down and shook hands with all the men in hospital, wishing them a happy day, and then they sent down a large sugared cake and some chocolate for the men who were well enough to enjoy it, and the very sick ones all had some champagne; the men appreciated it very much, and there was a great demand for envelopes to take "a bit of Bobs' cake home."

Many of the beautiful baskets of flowers that came on board for Lady Roberts at the different ports found their way down to the hospital, and the men especially treasured a beautiful Union Jack that came on board at Madeira, made of red geraniums and blue and white violets.

By the 22nd it had become cooler and rather damp, so all the men returned to the hospital (from the upper deck). On the 24th one of the officer patients had to have an anæsthetic for a slight operation on his arm; and I had a busy night in the hospital, as one man had a fit, and there were several enterics very ill.

On Christmas Day it was good to see about twenty officers and between forty and fifty men at the early Communion Service, and we also had a service in the hospital. The saloon was quite full for the morning services at 9.15 and at 10 A.M.—there were too many for all to attend one service.

Sister and I found two huge stockings on our plates at breakfast time, with all sorts of silly presents in them. We had a very pleasant day and a jolly dinner party at night.

We reached Madeira that evening, and did not leave again till 2 P.M. the next day, so I had a run ashore with some people in the morning. On the 28th we anchored at Gibraltar at 8.30 A.M., and the guns thundered out such a welcome to Lord Roberts! We stayed there till 1 P.M. the next day, and I again went ashore with some friends, and had a good look round the town.

Sir George White and his daughter came on board, and afterwards Lord and Lady Roberts went ashore.

We had fairly good weather all the way home, but after Gibraltar the ship was rather inclined to roll; the remark on the ship's log was "fresh to moderate gale, with confused (!) sea." Two of the sisters were rather bad, so the remaining sister and I had a busy time between the sick officers and the hospital; and, though neither of us was sea-sick, I can't say that we exactly enjoyed it when we had to sponge a bad typhoid in an upper berth (to reach whom we had to stand on a box, and have a man wedged in the gangway to hold our basin of water; never quite sure whether the next roll would not oblige him to pitch all the water over either us or our patient); and the daily syringing of the arm of the officer who had the operation was just about as much as I could stand on the rough days; so we were glad when the wind abated, and all the sisters could take their turn for night duty, &c.

Lord Roberts was awfully nice to me about having looked after the men on board, and he asked me whether I wanted anything he could help me with; so I told him I only wanted to be sure they would let me go back and do some more work, and not get sent to a home station; so he most kindly sent for his secretary, and asked him to write to the Director-General to say he would be obliged if my wishes on this point could be attended to. Was it not kind of him? If I had not been so surprised I should have asked to be allowed to work for the same Major again, but he was just chatting in such a kind, informal way on the deck, that I did not realise how much he could have helped me if I had thought to ask.

I saw the New Year in down in the hospital, and the stokers made such a noise to celebrate it, beating with their shovels, &c. Luckily, by then, all our patients were improving, though some of them were still very ill; all except the very sick ones were tremendously excited at the thought of getting home.

We were rather before our time, so, on the evening of January 1st, we had to anchor in Swanage Bay, and then arrived and anchored off Cowes the next morning at 10 A.M. It was freezing hard and bitterly cold, and we were all longing to get home; but in the afternoon Lord Roberts went ashore to be received by Queen Victoria at Osborne. He returned an Earl and a Knight of the Garter, and I believe the Queen handed him the V.C. won by his son at Colenso.

That night we anchored off Netley, and the cold was intense; we got up to Southampton at 9.30 A.M. on January 3rd, and such a crowd was there to welcome Lord Roberts. Of course it was some time before he got away and we could get our patients landed; but as soon as we got into dock some orderlies came on board from Netley with a good supply of fresh milk, which was much enjoyed in the hospital, and, eventually, we were thankful to see all the bad cases safely off to Netley—three of them had been so very ill, and several times we had thought they could not live to get home.

It is always a little sad saying good-bye to people you have got to know well on board ship, but not nearly so bad near home as out at the front.

We had orders to report ourselves at the War Office, and, after having cleared up the hospital, we were able to get away about 1 P.M.

The next day I called at the War Office, and presented Lord Roberts' letter, and was told that I should go back; they would let me know when—and then I went on leave.

On the 15th of January I had a wire to rejoin the ship for the return voyage on the 19th. It was bitterly cold all the time I was in England, and I had rather a rush to get some new uniform and other necessaries, to unpack and "sort myself," and repack again.

When I got on board the *Canada* I was rejoiced to find that Sister —— was returning too, and three of our original medical officers.

The ship was very full (122 in the saloon), and there were sixteen sisters and one other lady; but my old friend, the stewardess, was kind enough to manœuvre so that I got a small cabin to myself.

Just before we got away the *Manhattan* backed into our stern, and sent us first with such a bang against the wharf, that the people standing there fell down flat like ninepins (and it was raining, so there were inches of mud for them to fall into!); and then we broke away from our moorings, with some visitors and the embarkation officers still on board. After a little excitement they managed to anchor off Netley, and found our damage was chiefly to the boat deck (one boat was stove in) and the railings—it would have been more serious if our steam had not been up and ready for us to get away, so they were able to get her under control at once—but there we had to remain all the next day repairing, and it was very tantalising having to waste that time on board, especially as I have some relations who live within a couple of miles of where we were anchored.

Before we sailed we heard that the Queen was very ill, and I fear she has been very feeble lately, and very much troubled about the war; so we all feel anxious, and every night when the band plays "God Save the Queen," and all stand at the salute, we wonder how she is.

XLI

S.S. "VICTORIAN" (between CAPE TOWN and DURBAN), *February 1901*.

Just as we got in sight of St. Helena on February 2nd our engines broke down, and we had to lay to for some hours while they were being repaired.

Then, as we steamed slowly up to the anchorage, H.M.S. *Thetis* signalled to us that our Queen had died on January 22nd; so we ought to have been singing "God Save the *King*" for the past eleven days.

The men were all joking and playing games, &c., when the news came, and then there was such a hush of sorrow on the boat, and all the games were put away. We were at St. Helena all the next day while the repairs were going on. The *Mongolian* arrived with 600 Boer prisoners, and last week they had 1300 from Simon's Town. Since we were last here some of the prisoners had made an attempt at escape, and they had also had a nasty mutiny amongst the men of the West Indian Regiment, who were stationed there.

We anchored in Table Bay, after a very uneventful voyage (with no work in the hospital, except five cases of German measles), on February 8th, but did not get alongside till the following evening; and then (as we were receiving fresh orders about every half hour) we stayed quietly on board till the 11th —when the *Canada* was sailing again.

The only thing that was definite was that the medical officers and sisters who had been in Natal before were to return to that command, but how to get there was a different matter; the ship by which they proposed to send us by was not yet in, and it seemed likely that when the *Canada* left we should remain on the wharf sitting on our boxes.

Sister —— and I were the only sisters who had been in Natal before, so we saw the others off by train for Pretoria and Elandsfontein.

Then the *City of Vienna* came in, and she was so full she could only just take on the medical officers, and Sister and I had to wait to go by some other boat; but we were told we could go out to Wynberg and lodge at the hospital till they could find berths for us, leaving our heavy baggage in store at the docks.

There we were kept waiting ten days for a ship, and had a very dull time of it, as we were afraid to go to any distance in case any sudden orders came for us.

Wynberg is a very pretty place in pine woods; but the huts were infested with creatures, so that sleep was difficult, and though we are neither of us very particular about our food, it was so badly served and dirty that we could not enjoy it.

I can't understand about the mess, as the sisters have to pay all their allowance of 21s. a week for food, and don't get anything like such good food as we had at a cost of 14s. or 15s. a week (though the actual cost of food is less at Cape Town), and they have no variety. There were some Pretoria sisters staying there to recruit after enteric, and I felt so sorry for them, as the food was absolutely unsuitable for convalescents; and they told me they had been very well cared for all the time they were ill at Pretoria, and so they were missing the careful feeding they had been used to.

Of course we did not get to know really very much about the hospital, as we were not on duty, and were only "lodgers," but a sister who came out with us was on duty, and was not at all happy; there were so many petty rules for the sisters that they seemed to spend their time in trying to evade them—not a good hospital tone.

We found no news at all in the Cape Town papers, but certainly the war does not seem likely to be over just yet; they say all civil traffic and mails north of De Aar have been stopped.

There was a rumour that there were Boers within thirty miles of Cape Town, so all the Boer prisoners were being sent away from Simon's Town. Some naval guns have been mounted on the "Lion's Head" (a part of Table Mountain), and the Town Guard were sent up there in watches, as well as some of the regulars.

The Town Guard were most energetic and constantly drilling. One day I wanted to speak to one of the Customs' men, and found they were all drilling with their rifles in the Customs' shed, and the Customs' business had to wait.

Then, of course, you will have heard there was plague in Cape Town, and there was some alarm lest it should get amongst the soldiers, and cripple us in that way; but they seem to be attacking it in an energetic way, and so far it is practically confined to the coloured people.

As usual it started among the rats on the South Arm at the docks; large numbers of them died, and the rest went off in a body to Green Point, at which place there is a large military camp, so that the sanitary officials were rather anxious.

Then the natives got frightened, and wanted to go home; but the Government stopped that by not allowing any of them to travel by train, except with special permits; this was partly to prevent their spreading the plague about the country, and also because it would have been difficult to get the dock work done if the natives had cleared.

At the same time a large native location is being built on the Cape flats (where they will all have to live), and a light railway to bring them into their work.

Rats are being bought for threepence each, and several hundreds of their bodies are being cremated daily at the gasworks.

At last we went into Cape Town and saw the P.M.O., but he said he could not say when we should get on; so we went on to our friend the embarkation officer, and told him that if there was no transport coming soon, we would pay our own passage to go up to Natal by a mailboat rather than waste more time at Wynberg; but he promised we should get a ship before the next mail and save our money, which we were glad enough to do; but my private opinion is that we should have been waiting at Wynberg still if we had not gone into Cape Town and agitated about it!

We paid a visit to the Yeomanry Hospital at Maitland, where a brother of Sister's was in as a patient (but getting better), and I found several old friends on the staff there.

At last, on the 20th, we received orders to join the *Victorian* at Cape Town. It was pouring with rain, but Sister —— went off at once to find a cab, while I hastily packed up, paid our mess bill, &c. Before she got back, there was a telephone message to tell us to hurry, as the ship was going soon; we bundled our things on to the cab, and just managed to catch a train at Wynberg, which (by good luck) was an express, as most of the trains loiter about at all the suburban stations.

At Cape Town we hastily cabbed to the P.M.O.'s office for orders, but were told to go straight down to the ship; at the dock gates I sent Sister on with our small things to the ship, to say we were coming, while I went to the agents, and was lucky in finding an empty trolley, and getting them to tumble our heavy baggage on to it, though they said it was too late for the *Victorian*, as she had been hooting for some time; however, I got on to the waggon and rattled down to the South Arm. There I found Sister —— looking very melancholy, as they told her on board we were not expected, and there was no room for us, and "where were our written orders?"

Of course we *had* no written orders, as all had been by telephone; but I did not mean to be left behind, so, taking my bag, and telling Sister to bring hers, I bundled up the gangway, which they were on the point of removing, and asked to see the C.O., telling them that I did not mind a bit if there was no cabin, but that we could travel on deck! Just then the embarkation officer came bustling along, and said that he had thought we could not get down in time, but that it was all right, and they had got to make room for us! So some soldiers soon carried our baggage on board, and as our last box came on the embarkation officer went off, and we were away.

The cabins were really all full, but, after some delay, two poor young officers had to double in with some others and give us their cabin.

The *Victorian* is rather a grubby boat—a cattle-boat when she is at home. There are two hundred Boer prisoners on board, going up to a place near Ladysmith; four of them are officers, who are berthed on the upper deck, but don't mess with us. They seem quite a superior sort (one of them was a Commandant), and they are very polite to us, always ready to move our chairs, or to do anything to help us.

There are about twenty officers in the saloon, and one officer's wife.

The ship is not accustomed to having any ladies on board, but every one is very good to us, and the stewards are most attentive (there is no stewardess).

I sit next to the C.O., a Colonel from Australia, who had had a bad fall from his horse, and is going back to Australia for the voyage to recruit (this boat is going to take time-expired men from Durban to Australia, and will return with a full load of men and horses from there); he and his son have both been fighting out here.

Just lately he has been a patient in the hospital where we have been lodging, and he speaks very plainly about the bad management there, after he had been very well nursed in another hospital up-country.

There is a very pleasant, and very Irish, R.A.M.C. Major in medical charge. He has had a rough time trekking about with his regiment for the last fifteen months, and is now going for the trip to Australia to recruit after fever; he wants us to go with him, as they will probably send a couple of sisters, and we already have the promise of "a good time" in Australia while the ship is there; Sister says she would like to go, but I would like to see this show through first.

The officer's wife has been in her cabin sea-sick all the way, so we have had to look after her a bit. It has been a little rough, but even Sister —— has kept well—we conclude because we had been doing a compulsory fast in consequence of the bad feeding at Wynberg before we came on board! We should have thought the feeding on this boat very poor after the *Canada*, but it is first rate after Wynberg.

We shall soon be at Durban now, and then they say we may have to be quarantined outside for ten days (on account of the plague at the Cape), but we hope our services may be so urgently required at the front that they may forget to quarantine us!

XLII

We arrived at Durban on February 23rd, and were eventually allowed to land without being quarantined.

It was Saturday afternoon, and no orders came on board for us, and by the time the Boer prisoners were landed, and we were able to get our baggage ashore, the Durban P.M.O. had left his office; so we felt free to do as we pleased till the following day, when (though Sunday) we *might* be able to report ourselves.

If we had been new sisters arriving it might have been awkward, but it suited us down to the ground.

Sister —— just caught the evening train up to Pinetown to stay with some friends, and I promised to wire to her if we were needed on Sunday; otherwise she would return on Monday.

Then a kind sergeant-major helped me to get our baggage on to a trolley and take it up to the medical store, where it would be quite safe; and after that I went up to see some friends on the Berea, and they most kindly took me in.

From them I learnt many things; amongst others, that our old hospital had been turned into a Rest Camp of 300 beds, and that they thought we were to have the chance of going back there, but, for various reasons, they strongly advised us not to do so if we could avoid it; that our late medical officers had already been sent farther up-country (we had hoped to work for them again, but did not succeed in doing so).

On Sunday morning I went to report "ourselves" to Major ——, and he was very pleasant and kind, wanted to hear all about our voyage home, &c., and asked me where we wanted to go? So I told him "as near up to the front as we could get"; then he told me that the order from the Natal P.M.O. was for us to return to Pinetown, but if I liked he would wire to him to ask him to let us go up-country, and that we could stay with our friends till he got a reply.

I had a quiet Sunday in Durban, meeting many friends, and going to church in the evening.

The next morning I met Sister at the station, and the first thing she said to me (before I could tell her the orders) was, "Sister, I *won't* go to Pinetown, I would rather resign, if they want to send us there." So then I told her that our fate was waiting on a wire from the P.M.O.; and as we walked along to the office she told me a good deal of what she had heard about Pinetown—of course we can scarcely judge how much of it is really true, but at any rate it appears that some of the sisters now there seem to think that they have come out to South Africa only to enjoy themselves, and that they are setting about it in a way which no lady would care to emulate.

It was rather strange that we should both have received the same advice from quite different sources: "Don't go there."

Together we went to the office, and stayed there some time, but no wire had come; they thought we should probably go *somewhere* by the 6 P.M. mail train. We were advised to take some food if we went up, as meals on the way were uncertain. So I stocked my tea-basket, and bought some potted meat, &c., in case we went.

All day we had to hover near the office or within sound of the telephone, and at 5 P.M. a wire came for us to go up to No. —— General Hospital by the mail train.

One of the medical officers kindly helped us to get our baggage to the station, and secured a carriage for us.

It is always a shaky journey up from Durban, but we got some sleep, and the next morning, when we were having breakfast at Glencoe, we were delighted to meet Major ——, of the Royal Engineers, an old patient of ours, who has done splendid work up this side; he was going down to Ladysmith.

A little farther on we met two officers who had come out in the *Canada* with us, so they came into our carriage, and shared our lunch, and we brewed some tea with my tea-basket. At Newcastle General Hilliard was on the platform, and also a sister whom we knew.

We had no sooner reached our destination than Sergeant C. came up to welcome us—he had been at Pinetown—and also went home with us; he does not seem at all pleased at being sent here, and is already trying to get a change.

This hospital has been a "Stationary Hospital" up to now, but is just being turned into a "General Hospital," so they say it is in rather a muddle at present.

Sister —— and I were allotted a tent with just bed and blankets—nothing else; we were not required on duty that day, so we went down to the coolie store and invested in some cheap sheets, a bucket, basin, &c.; also table fittings, as they told us no plates, cups, knives, or anything were provided. Many people out here prefer to sleep in blankets, but as the army blankets are dark brown, rather of the texture of horsecloths, and as these were obviously not new (and the washing and disinfecting of army blankets in a satisfactory way is still an unsolved problem out here), we preferred to put some sheets in between!

The air is lovely and fresh up here, where we are 5000 feet above the sea-level—always hot sun in the day, but very cold nights.

A most unfortunate thing occurred the first night we were here: a sister, who came out in the *Canada* with us, had two large cases of feather cushions given her by the Princess of Wales—whom we must now learn to call Queen Alexandra—with the request that they should go to men in hospital near up to the front. She had promised me that if I went up-country I should have one of the boxes to distribute.

When we arrived here I found a wire from her saying that she was passing our station about 8.30 P.M., and would I meet her? She was one of the sisters who had landed at Cape Town, but was now coming down to a hospital on this side. So, when we had got our tent straight, we went to the Lady Superintendent and said that if we were really not wanted on duty, might we go down to the station after dinner to meet this sister? She said certainly we might; she was sorry she had some letters to write, or she would have walked down with us.

When we got to the station we found we were rather too soon, and there were a lot of orderlies standing about, and a few officers (whom, of course, we did not know), so I said to Sister, "I vote we walk about outside till we hear the train coming"; and we were just beating a retreat from the platform when an officer stalked up and said, in a very rude way, "Who are you?" We just gave our names, and were walking away, when he again stopped us, and asked what we wanted at the station? By this time Sister —— was bubbling over with wrath, but we had to explain that we had obtained leave to meet a sister. I believe if I had said that I was expecting a box of things from the Queen, he would have knuckled under, but I was not going to trade on that; and the long and short of it was that he did not believe that we had been given leave, and said we were not allowed in the station and were to return to camp.

Of course we went back furious at his rudeness, and then discovered he was the C.O. here! I expect the Lady Superintendent had forgotten to tell him we had leave (or something of that kind), but he might have believed our word, and not been so rude to us before a lot of orderlies, and she was very much annoyed with him.

The next morning, when we were formally introduced to him, he was, I think, penitent, and invited us to go out for a picnic on the following day, when some people whom we knew were coming here, partly to inspect the hospital and partly for this excursion. Sister —— went with them, but I was going on night duty that night, so I begged off.

This is a "Ration Station" (as it would be difficult to buy food privately so far from the base), therefore we don't get quite so many "allowances," but the "skoff" seems very fairly good; they bake bread in the camp; and as long as you can get decent bread you can be content.

We are just on the border of the Transvaal, and there are plenty of Boers about; two or three of our columns are trekking about in the district, and they say that we often have sick and wounded sent in from them.

Most of the sisters here seem to ride, but I can't take to that again yet. The night sisters had a little excitement two nights ago, when two horses galloped into the camp, and they—with the help of a convalescent officer—caught and tethered them. They hoped they would be allowed to keep them, but, unfortunately, they were reclaimed by some Yeomanry men; but they say that very often droves of horses pass here, and sometimes a few escape, or are left behind too sick (or too tired) to go on; and then the orderlies catch them and sell them to the sisters for £1 or £2!

I think there are about 500 beds here, nearly all under canvas. There are a few buildings of wood, and amongst them is a small room that the sisters use as a duty room, and the night sisters (two of them) sit there, and they have a small stove for boiling water, &c. There is no arrangement for hot water near the tents for the patients—we used to have (and I have seen them in other hospitals too) boilers on wheels with a coolie to keep the fire going, and if the water was not always hot, the coolie soon heard about it from the orderlies.

One day the C.O. asked me whether I had everything I wanted, and I said, "No, I wanted a good many things for the men, one being hot water"; but he said he had never heard of these movable boilers, and seemed to think them an unnecessary luxury.

At the sisters' camp we have a comfortable room that they use as a sitting-room, with a mixed lot of furniture that has been "commandeered" from houses in the district. The other day an officer sent us a lot of china plates taken from a Boer hotel; they were very welcome, as we were most of us using enamel plates out of our tea-baskets, &c. We have our meals in a tent —just a long table, and benches without backs.

Our sleeping tents are chiefly the big square kind, called E. P. tents; they are supposed to hold four beds, so we may have to pack tight, but at present Sister and I are alone. Some of the sisters have made their tents very nice, and have rigged up curtains to divide them. At present we use our boxes as washstand, &c., and as a General Hospital is given a certain amount of furniture for the sisters, we intend not to buy anything that is not really necessary until we see what they are going to give us.

XLIII

Now I have waded (both literally and figuratively) through my first spell of a fortnight on night duty, and it has not been pleasant; but when one thinks how much worse it must be for the troops out trekking, one does not mind.

I have always thought that South Africa *without the sun* was rather a poor sort of a place, and, living in a tent in the wet season, I am confirmed in that opinion.

It began to rain the first night I went on duty, and during the fortnight I had only four fine nights: the other nights it rained—generally in bucketfuls.

The first day when I went to bed it was very hot and stuffy in the tent, so I did not sleep for some time, but was sleeping in the afternoon when the rain began, and soon it woke me up by splashing on my face; then I found it was coming down in torrents, and our tent had been so badly pitched, with no trench round it, that there was a deep stream flowing through. I had to paddle about and rescue all our goods from the floor, pitching most of them on to Sister's bed; and she was rather amused when she came over to call me, to find me fast asleep under a mackintosh and umbrella, my bed a simple island, and no room for her to get into her own bed!

Most of the sisters were prepared for this, and had suitable garments, but it was several days before I could obtain them, so I very soon had not a dry garment to my name.

Before I leave the subject I may as well tell you what is the correct garb, and then you can imagine us sitting on a bench at our mess—and I am sure no one seeing us would think we were sisters; with our lanterns hung up behind us, we look more like miners, or something of that sort!

The first essential is a pair of knee "gum" boots, as the grass between the tents is long; then you must have knickerbockers, with a very short serge skirt (some omit the skirt altogether on night duty!), then a mackintosh. When it does not rain, you substitute for the mackintosh a "British Warmer" coat—that is the short khaki overcoat that both officers and privates wear, a very rough wool with a warm flannel lining. For headgear we have a sailor hat, or a wool cap, or a sou'wester, according to taste. White caps and aprons are quite impossible when you have to go from tent to tent.

Of course there is no chance of drying anything till the sun comes out again, and when we get out of bed it would never do to turn it down; instead of that you put anything you wish to *try* to keep dry inside, and cover it all up with every rug and blanket and mackintosh that you can lay hands on.

Our tent was so hopelessly bad, that after some days they let us move into another, and that one having a wooden floor, we were better off.

I was so tired after moving our things into the new tent, and after a heavy night on duty in the pouring rain, that I slept like a top, and when I woke in the evening I found everything upset in the tent, and evident marks that a cow had been taking shelter with me!

The sisters gibed at me, and said I should probably not have waked up if it had been a Boer commando.

There are a lot of men very ill. I was supposed to have charge on night duty of the medical side (about 250 beds), and that included the enteric tents with about 100 beds. They seem to have a mania for shifting the men about, so it was often difficult to find the bad cases; there were generally only night orderlies in the enteric tents, so that men who needed much attention in the night were supposed to be sent to the enteric line, whether they had enteric or not. To escape this risk of infection for them, we sisters used to try to do all for them in their own tents as long as we possibly could, and the poor chaps were so grateful to us, and the day sisters (who were equally keen not to have them sent down) used to tell us that the men always assured the medical officers that they had everything they wanted in the night. You know how at home if a sick man wakes up, and is alone for a few minutes, he thinks he is being neglected, but these poor chaps must have many lonely hours in the dark tents, and yet they never complain; they know that so many are dying of enteric, and they seem to have a horror of being sent down to that line.

It really was pretty horrid paddling about in the dark and the long grass between the tents; and it was so slippery with mud and rain that twice I fell down, and it took some time before I could find my lantern and the kettle which I had just boiled up, and was carrying down to make a poultice for a poor chap with pneumonia: it was very annoying, as, of course, it took time to reboil the kettle. The day sister leaves everything ready, with the linseed in a bowl, so that I have only to pour the water on, and then I put everything all ready for the next one; in this way we can get fairly hot poultices, though the tents are a long way from the fire.

The men used to be so sorry for us being so constantly wet; and many a convalescent man used to beg me to let him stay awake with a man who was very ill and give him his drinks, &c., promising to come and fetch me if he wanted anything, so that I need not go round so often,—but, of course, I could not let him do that.

One man (a New Zealander) said to me, "Well, Sister, I have often grumbled at having to do sentry-go for two or three hours on a wet night, but I never knew that any woman had to do it for twelve hours at a stretch; I shan't grumble at my share again in a hurry."

The other day we had in a big convoy of eighty sick and wounded from General French's column. They had been eight days in ox waggons coming seventy-two miles; poor chaps, they were glad to get into beds.

Two days from here they had got stuck in a drift one night, and the Boers came down and fired on them, killing a corporal and a private of the guard and wounding two others. One man had been shot in the thigh, and Sister made him comfortable in bed, and the doctor said they should not do anything till next day; the man slept like a top for over twelve hours, and when he woke in the morning Sister said something to him about having been comfortable, and he said, "Yes, Sister, I was not going to miss five minutes' enjoyment of that bed, for I have not been on a bed for fifteen months."

This convoy also brought in a lot of Boer women and children, but they have gone into a camp about three miles from here.

If you, or any of your friends, care to post me any illustrated papers or magazines, they would be most gratefully received, or in fact anything wherewith to amuse the men. We should be very glad, too, of warm garments, as the winter is coming on, and the Red Cross people have stopped sending the splendid big bundles of papers that our men used to appreciate so much; in fact, most people seem to have tired of sending the things with which we were so well supplied at first. The poor Tommies feel a little hurt at no free supplies of tobacco or cigarettes, and I would give anything to have my old supply of warm shirts, sweaters, wool caps, &c., for the men who have to go back to roughing it on trek.

Now that the rain has stopped, we are having perfectly lovely days, but the nights are very cold; they say that a little later on it is bitterly cold up here.

There were six deaths during my first fortnight on night duty, and it was awfully sad, as one felt they had so little chance, and I cannot really see why they should not be better "done by"; but the sisters seem to think that it is the natural order of things, and that we must just "do our best and leave the rest."

The General was here the other day, and said that all the men were to have tumblers instead of mugs, but I suppose he does not know that they have not each got a mug yet!

There is one enteric tent (the last one opened) of fourteen beds, and their equipment includes only four mugs, and not a single feeding-cup at all. One night I found a man, who had not got enteric, sent there for the sake of having night orderlies, as he was very ill; so I had to borrow a mug for him from another line, and the next day I bought him the necessary fittings at the coolie store; but it won't do much good, as the orderlies probably won't take proper precautions to wash up for him separately.

There are some new R.A.M.C. officers here now, and one of them seems energetic; I don't know what had gone wrong that he was poking into, but one of the sisters heard him say to a sergeant, "Hospital scandals are not in it," so we can only hope things will improve here.

There was much excitement here one night. A major arrived, sick, in a mule buggy from a column near here; the C.O. saw him, and told him what tent to go to, but he never arrived. After much searching of the camp, neither the officer nor his mules could be found; then the heliograph was set to work, and eventually he was located at the next station, and when he was brought back he said the C.O. was so rude to him that he thought he would not stay, and had gone to a hotel!

Since I came off night duty I, and two other sisters, have been doing only "afternoon duty," which means looking after the camp while all the other sisters are off duty; this is because there are more sisters here than the proper number: if there were only the right number, two of the sisters who have lines would stay on every afternoon in turn; but the stupid thing about it is that if we were each turned on to a big tent of enterics (instead of one sister having all the line on her hands) we might be doing really useful nursing; as it is, there is not much to do in the afternoon, beyond prowling round and trying to talk to the men and cheer them up a bit.

The other day one of them presented me with these lines of his own composition; he was in a tent when I was on night duty where there was a very bad case:

(*By an Australian Trooper.*)

You may talk of our Soldiers and Sailors,
   Of our brave Colonials too,
But nothing is thought of our Nurses,
   With hearts so tender and true.

They have suffered great hardships, and endured
   The trials that fell to their share,
And so caused their names to be cherished
   On every Barrack Room Square.

So give three cheers for our Sisters
   Who've shown us what they will do
To help the cause of Old England
   By nursing our sick soldiers through.

XLIV

Our tent has filled up now—four of us in it—so we feel rather tightly packed. One of the four is a sister who has been in India, and done some camping out, so she thinks she knows all about tents and how to live in them; we rather trade on this, and when it rains we assure her she ought to go round and slack the guy-ropes in case they should shrink with the wet and pull the pegs up, as she knows so much more about how to do it than we do; or if it comes on to blow in the night we wake her up, and offer her the hammer to go round and knock in the tent-pegs!

The wind gets up so suddenly here that we have to be careful not to leave anything about that is not tethered, or it may be miles away over the veldt before we wake up.

I now have charge of a medical line of tents, and find the work very interesting, though there are many difficulties to contend with.

The Boers seem very thick in the country round; they have captured a train with 250 horses between here and H., and the other day they took 600 head of cattle from a loyal farmer only about six miles from here, and he had to fly for protection.

Some Dragoons, who have been scouring the country for some weeks, were through here the other day, and one of their poor horses fell, exhausted, near to my tent; after a rest they got him up and went on, but soon a sergeant returned to say that he had fallen again, and they were going to shoot him, could he borrow some mules and tackle to pull his body off the path? I said, "Oh, don't shoot him—I badly want a horse, and I'll get him some gruel and brandy from the store." He said I might have him if I would look after him, or else get him shot; but when we went out we found the men had already shot the poor beast.

There are so many dead horses, mules, and oxen about that it is rather horrid walking anywhere beyond the camp, and sometimes we hear that the Boers have put a dead mule (and once we heard some dead Kaffirs) into our water supply, and it makes us rather squeamish, as we can't even get our drinking water boiled here. Some of the officer patients tell us that they have drunk nothing but boiled water all through the campaign until they came here, and now they can't get it boiled for them.

I am beginning to get papers from home, and they are much appreciated by the men, especially the six numbers of the *Daily Mail* that come each week; I take one to each of my tents, and then they exchange them about. Of course they are a month old, but, for all that, they are the latest news, and heaps of men from other lines congregate to hear them read.

After much trouble I have retrieved that box of cushions sent by the Queen, and they are treasures indeed; nice big feather cushions covered in red twill, and labelled "A present from the Princess of Wales." It was a little difficult to know to whom to give them, as, of course, all the men wanted one. I am trying to give them to invalids who will go home when well enough, as they will be very useful on the voyage, and the men could hardly carry them with them on trek.

We had much excitement here early this month: one morning we were awakened at 5 A.M. by the sound of big guns, and in the course of time we heard that the Boers had blown up some culverts in the night, and captured a provision train; then there was a heliograph message to say, "Heavy fighting since daybreak," and they wanted some medical officers; so two men went off with ambulances, but it seems none of our men were wounded; five or six Boers were killed, and two of their wounded were brought here: one poor chap with a shell wound of the head is not likely to live; he looked just a rough country boy in corduroys, but he has "F. J. Joubert" marked on a handkerchief, so he may be some relation of the General.

The guard of the train had a rough time, as they took away his boots, and then made him carry sacks of provisions for them up a steep kopje.

For the present, they have stopped the trains from running at night. I do think the railway men have been awfully plucky in sticking to their work, when they could never feel confident that the line was not mined.

We had orders not to go outside the camp for some days, and the C.O. went round and took notes of all the men who were fit to take a rifle if there was an attack; and of course all the men ride about armed.

We had a quiet Easter Day here. The sisters were expecting some officers of the 5th Dragoons over to tea, but they did not turn up, as they had been out all night chasing Boers.

A few days later the Boers burnt a hotel and stores at Ingogo, and some troops were hurried through here to go after them, but of course they got away.

Still a great many deaths here; the other day we had four in twenty four hours; one of those who died was a doctor whom I knew slightly (he travelled up the coast with us when we first came out). He had been practising out here, so his wife was able to come and be with him, and she stayed in our camp. The poor man had heart disease. Of course he wasn't in my line, but the sister of the officers' ward had a case in the theatre, and as he had been asking for me the Lady Superintendent asked me if I would go to sit with him if I could leave my line for a bit. I managed to be with him most of the day, and he died in the evening, and I went with his wife to the funeral the next day.

The enteric line is now full, so one of my tents has been allowed to have night orderlies, and we collect the bad cases into that.

You would be amused at a "kit inspection" here: when one is proclaimed, the excitement is great, and the orderlies, almost tearing their hair, are so distracted that if the sister has any bad cases, she must nurse them herself, or understand that they will get no attention till the inspection is over! All the ward equipment, mugs, plates, buckets, brooms, &c., has to be laid out at the tent door for the officers to count. In a hospital at home, when "stock-taking" comes, you know that anything that is worn out, or damaged, or really lost, will be replaced, and you are glad of the chance of getting things made correct; but here they assure me that things must *be* correct, or the orderly gets fined or punished; so, to avoid this, he resorts to strategy.

As soon as the officer (with the wardmaster and orderly in attendance) has passed one tent as correct, the things may be put away again, and then comes in the help of the patients (who fully enter into the game), the most nimble trotting off with a medicine glass to one orderly who is short of that, or a bucket to another; I have known a good broom do duty for three different lines by careful dodging about.

I find one of the senior sisters here is one who applied to me when I was choosing sisters to bring out at first; but I had many to choose from, and I made no mistake in thinking others more suited for the work! Another sister who *did* come out with me has recently come up here, but she has not been very well since she came, and thinks the life here is very rough, so she is trying to get an exchange.

Sisters can get away from here only by inducing others to exchange with them; and it is not easy to make any one believe that this is a desirable station. I have not tried yet, as I want to stick to it if I can (of course I can't do much, but I can make a few men more comfortable), but most of the others are trying to exchange.

Our meat chiefly consists of trek ox, and it is so tough that it is difficult to tackle; about once a week we get skinny mutton.

The bread is all right, but several times lately the butter has not arrived, and we have to do without. We buy chocolates and biscuits at the coolie store to fill up the cracks.

The other day we had in a sick convoy that had been seven days on the road, and one poor fellow was so bad with dysentery that he died an hour after they lifted him out of the ambulance; really these long days of knocking about in the ambulances seem about the worst of the hardships that the poor chaps have to put up with, especially for the very sick or the wounded. You see, most of the waggons are drawn by about sixteen mules, and sometimes they trot and sometimes they walk, but sometimes they turn really mulish and won't budge; and then, after much hauling and thrashing and shouting, they start with a great bound and go off at a gallop. They are seldom on anything that you could call a road, and are much more frequently on the rough veldt.

A man who has been badly wounded can tell you all about the day when he got knocked over—he does not care to say much about the long day in the blazing sun, when he lay thirsty where he fell before the Bearer Company came along; and then, perhaps, the dark night with frost on the ground, or rain falling; he shudders when he tells you of the groaning men who lay around him, and who gradually ceased to groan, and how he began to think the ambulance would be too late to pick him up too—but what he simply can't bear to speak about is the agony of being pitched about with a fractured bone for days in one of those waggons.

It is not so bad when the fighting is anywhere near the rail, as then the wounded are soon placed in the hospital trains, and are fairly comfortable; but the long days of travelling by waggon are terrible.

General Dartnell's column was through here the other day, and they have gone into camp about two miles from us for ten days' rest. He has about 3000 men with him, and they have about filled us up with sick, while a good many went straight on board a hospital train.

Major ——, of the Commander-in-Chief's Bodyguard, was with this column, and came over to see me; his wife was in Cape Town when I was last there, and went home on the *Canada*. You know how particular he is about his horses, &c., at home? He drove over to see me in a very ramshackle old Cape cart with a big horse running as a pair with a rough little Boer pony. His uniform was in rags, and we did a little stitching up for him before he returned; they are having a very rough time of it.

XLV

There have been some big ructions here lately, but I think, perhaps, they may have done good in some ways.

I don't think that I told you of a difficulty with which I had to wrestle when I was on night duty, and which bothered me a good deal.

I believe it is a general rule in the Army Nursing Service that the sisters give all the medicines and stimulants; and, of course, I expected to do the same here, but when I got to the enteric line on night duty, I found that the day sister left them all to the orderlies to give in the daytime, and the night orderlies gave them in the night. Generally there were good orderlies there, who were quite to be trusted, but every now and then there were odd men on, and of course I could not be sure that the stimulants, &c., were correctly given. The day sister gave me no report of what the men were on, but it was given to the orderly.

I did not quite know what to do, but I went to the Lady Superintendent (after seeing the sister of the enteric line) and told her that if I was to be responsible that they were given, would she arrange that I was given the report, as otherwise I could not tell that everything was given as directed; but if it was right to leave it in the hands of the orderlies I would *try* to see that it was all right, but would not be responsible if anything went wrong. She seemed to think the day sister would not have time to give all herself (she had charge of only the one line, whereas the night sisters each had five or six lines). Anyhow, she did not do anything at all in the matter, so I just muddled on as best I could, and used always to try to be around when important medicines were due, so that I don't *think* much was neglected. Then, last month, another night sister was on, who did not get on well with the orderlies, and she reported one of them for being asleep, and he promptly replied by reporting her for not doing her duty and giving the medicines, &c., so that he had to do it all.

Then came the ructions, and now the sisters have to give everything, and I believe they are going to put on a third night sister, so I think things will go more smoothly in time.

The Lady Superintendent has only once been round my line since I have had charge of it.

I had a curious case the other day that gave us a good deal of anxiety—that of a young lance-corporal, who had been bad with malaria, but was better and able to sit up in bed. I left him one night very cheery and bright, and the next morning I happened to meet the night sister as she went off duty, and she said, "Oh, Sister, I forgot to report that that lance-corporal of yours in tent 3 did not seem so well, and he was sick this morning." I thought that I would go and look at him first instead of beginning my round in tent 1, and I was shocked to find the poor boy quite unconscious, and almost pulseless. Of course I sent for the doctor and got brandy, hot bottles, &c.; the doctor thought it was all up, but he injected strychnine; he said he thought it must have been typhoid and not malaria, and that this meant perforation. Anyhow, the boy began to revive; I hardly left him all day, but now I think I may say he is out of danger; I really think it was heart trouble, perhaps embolism, but I have seldom seen a man pull round after being as nearly gone as he was.

Of course you will have heard that the poor old *Tantallon Castle*, the ship on which we first came out, has gone down on Robben Island. The passengers and the mails were saved, and I was rejoiced when a nice, soft little blanket arrived that my people had sent out by her; I roll myself in it inside my sheets, and am much more comfortable.

It is a curious thing that so many ships in which I have travelled have gone to the bottom: I made one trip years ago up the coast on the *Drummond Castle*, and went down the coast on the *Courland Castle*; I also went home from Tenerife on the *Fez*—they have all gone down, and now the *Tantallon Castle* has shared their fate.

There was a big dance one night about three miles from here, to which twelve of the sisters went, and another night there were some theatricals. I daresay I am wrong, but somehow these festivities seem a little out of place while the war is still going on. Some of the sisters appear to think that they have come out here to have as much fun as they can get, and they talk about very little except the men they have been dancing with, and so on.

The wind has been tremendous lately, and four of the patients' tents have been blown to ribbons; we seem to spend most of our time on duty trying to keep the men's tents up (with not more of the gale than is absolutely necessary blowing round the bad cases), and most of our time off duty in attending to our own tent-pegs, &c. Of course wind here always means dust, and sometimes it seems as though the stones fly up and hit you in the face, and unless one takes great care the patients' milk is soon full of sand.

Really, if it was not that the men suffered for them, some of our difficulties would be amusing. When this hospital was a "Field Stationary" all the men had warm, grey flannel shirts; when it became a "General" they were given instead white cotton shirts and white flannel vests. That was all right at first, but recently the hospital has been enlarged, and, though there are plenty of the cotton shirts, they have run out of the flannel vests. Now the winter has begun, and we have many men in with rheumatism and chest complaints, and the tents are very cold, but the poor chaps are only given cotton shirts. I know there are plenty of the old "greybacks" in the store, but because this is now called a General Hospital they are not correct, and so cannot be issued, and the men must wait till more vests arrive! We have all fussed about it as much as we could, and we bought flannel shirts at the store for our worst cases (a man is always most grateful for an extra shirt to take with him when he goes away, so they won't be wasted), and now, at last, the old greybacks have been dealt out. At last they have got some boilers on wheels, so that we can get hot water in the tents; but *why* should we have to wrestle so long to get things that make so much difference to the health and the comfort of the men? The Lady Superintendent is always saying that she does not know how we should have done in Ladysmith; but we all reply that we should have tried to make shift, but we can't see why we should have to "make shift" here quite so much, with an open line to the base.

I do wonder when the war will be over: the poor Tommies are so heartily sick of it, and are beginning to try every means to get sent home; you see most of the excitement of war has pretty well worn off, and now they just have to keep on trekking about the country, destroying farms, and bringing in Boer women and children to the refugee camps. They generally collect more destitute people on the way than they reckoned for, and, as they have to feed them, the rations for the troops run short, and the men are cut down to half rations (and sometimes quarter rations); and some columns out this way have had nothing but "mealie meal" (Indian corn), and not too much of that, for some days before they got into camp. Sometimes they have been on such short rations that men have had to be punished for stealing their horses' rations of mealie meal. When they pass through a village, the first place they make for is the baker's shop, and it is very soon cleared, and you see the men going on with loaves slung around them, and rather in the way of their rifles. When you consider that they are generally marching all day in a hot sun, and that in summer the nights are often wet, and in winter they are generally frosty, and the men just have to lie down hungry on their mackintosh sheet (no tents), with their greatcoat and sometimes one blanket; that they hardly ever have a chance of shooting at a Boer, but are constantly being sniped at during the nights—is it any wonder that they are utterly weary of it all?

We have not heard so much about Boers being close around here since General Dartnell's column went through, and now the sisters are generally allowed to ride again.

Our tent is the last one at this end of the camp, and when we were told that we were not to go more than a mile from the camp in any direction (except along the line) it used to be strange to walk out, after we came off duty, for a few hundred yards beyond my tent, and then sit down on a grassy ridge as it got dark and watch the heliographs flashing around, and wonder whether the little lights we saw meant our men or Boers camping out. Sometimes we used to imagine they were quite close and watching us, and used to go back to our tents feeling quite creepy, and borrowing an extra piece of string to tie up our tent door!

And then, when we heard the guns in the distance, it was always a debatable point whether it was worth getting up and dressing in case any wounded were brought in soon, but we generally decided to finish our usual allowance of hours in bed.

People are kindly sending me English papers now, both from England and passed on from Durban, and they are very much enjoyed; the men were especially delighted last week when they got hold of an old weekly edition of *The Times* in which General Buller and General Roberts mentioned some of the regiments to which they belonged.

It is getting frightfully cold at nights; there are big icicles hanging round the water tanks, and when one of them overflowed there was quite a little sea of ice round it; the water in our tents often freezes, and it is quite difficult to break it to wash in the morning.

The night sisters are very miserable with the cold; I shall have to take my turn on night again next month, and I shall be quite sorry to give up my line, as the patients are so awfully grateful for what one can do for them, and I have nice orderlies just now.

We go to bed directly we finish dinner at night, so as to try to get warm.

XLVI

Thank goodness the winter will soon be over. I have never felt anything like the keenness of the cold up here.

On the whole, things have been fairly quiet in the country round just lately, though once the line was threatened and some of the trains delayed; and on another day there was a rumour of fighting not far off, and it was said that we had lost some guns, but I don't think there was much truth in the report.

Things are also going a little better in the hospital. We have a new Lady Superintendent, the other having gone home on a hospital ship.

There has been another big dance, to which most of the sisters went, and some other entertainments.

One night we (my tent full) had all gone to bed to try to get warm, when some one came banging on the canvas, and Sister —— of the Hospital Train put her head in; you know she was an old London friend of mine.

Her train was tied up here for the night, and, as she had heard our men were suffering from the cold, she had brought up a noble present of flannel jackets for them. They really were treasures: of course, I wanted them all for my own line, but had to be generous and give up a few to sisters who really had some bad chest and rheumatism patients.

Talking about rheumatism—I had one man in with rheumatism who was rather bad at first; he would not improve, but remained so helpless that the orderly had to lift him about. I did not quite know what to do with him, and began to think that if an R.A.M.C. surgeon had been on my line the improvement would have been rather more rapid than with the civil surgeon who had charge! Then, one day, I had a man bad in the next tent to this man, so I asked leave to go down to do something for him one evening after we had gone off duty, as I knew the night sister would be too busy to go to him when she first went on—and here there is always an hour's interval after the day sisters leave the camp and before the night sisters go down. What was my surprise when I got to the tent to find my rheumatic patient in there playing cards! He had pretended he could not sit up in bed.

I only said to him that I thought it was time he turned in for the night; and the next day I handed his board to the medical officer when he came round, and said that if he did not mind marking him "up," I thought it would do him good to sit out in the sun in the middle of the day, if the orderly put him to bed after tea. You can imagine the poor man felt pretty small, and in a few days he told the civil surgeon that he thought he felt fit to go back to duty, so we shook hands and parted good friends. I hope that he will not get shot, or I shall wish I had let him slack a bit longer!

We have had a good many Boer patients in lately; one poor young captain has lost his leg. One old fellow used to crawl about on crutches, but he was caught one night slipping about without them, and a Boer woman was found outside the fence with his clothes; so now all the Boers have been collected together and a guard posted.

I am now on night duty again, and find the orderlies more attentive, and the patients (generally) better nursed.

The first night I was on duty I was just reading the reports and trying to find out where the worst cases were, so as to visit them first (I now have 285 beds on my side, instead of the 250 I had when I was on before), when a wardmaster came to tell me that a sick convoy had turned up unexpectedly from General Bullock's column, and one man had been wounded on the way and had some hæmorrhage from a shattered hand. I helped the surgical sister get the theatre ready in a hurry, and then she stayed for the operation, while I went to see the others. There were only fifteen men, and they were black as sweeps and very cold; but they did not seem very bad, and they were delighted to be in shelter, with the prospect of a bed.

The orderly officer asked me to give them anything I liked, and he would order it afterwards, while he went to the theatre with the case; the wardmaster got them all some Bovril, and we soon settled which of them might have bread with it; and then I had not the heart to insist on the usual wash, as it was so bitterly cold, but I let them all tumble into beds, and then took round a bottle of whisky and a kettle and gave them all a hot drink; there was nothing more heard of that lot of men (but snores) for a good many hours! Poor chaps, they were absolutely tired out, and the medical officer quite approved, only saying he thought they might have had two bottles of whisky amongst them instead of one, but you know I am a strict teetotaller!

Having settled them, I started my rounds, and soon found that the worst case was a poor chap with pneumonia; fortunately he was in a building (instead of a tent), so it was possible to keep him fairly warm. The night orderly was not a very intelligent youth, but he was fairly watchful and obedient, and for four nights I spent every spare minute with this man, and really thought we should pull him through; then the fifth night the day sister met me in a very bad temper, and said, "What *do* you think? they have moved our poor O. down to a very draughty enteric tent; after all the trouble we have taken to pull him round! I am sure he will die there." I asked why he had been moved, as there had been no sign of enteric, and she replied that she could not get any reason, but an orderly had told her that "the doctor said that he was going to die, and he did not want any death up there."

Poor chap, he did die the next day, and of course he *might* have done so in any case, but to shift him then just took away his only chance.

It has been very cold all the time that I have been on night duty, but two of the nights were so horrible that I don't think I shall ever forget them. Sister —— is on with me now, so we grumble together; for those two nights it was blowing *hard*, and then a sleety rain came on that positively cut like knives, and was almost paralysing; on the second of those two nights I struggled back to the duty room and flopped down by the fire, which was very low, but I had not even the energy to poke it up; after a bit Sister came in dripping wet and looking blue with cold; she set down her lantern, and then came to the fire and gazed at me, and, after a bit, said, "Sister, you do look ill." I tried to laugh, but I think we were both much nearer crying with cold; so I struggled up to attend to the fire and brewed some tea, and after a bit Sister said, "Do you know, Sister, when I came in I thought you looked as though you were going to die, and if you had been, I positively had not the power to set to work to get you a hot drink or anything."

I told her I thought we were both too tough to die of cold, and then we both (feeling a little better for the tea and warmth) had to tramp off again to give brandy to some of the bad cases. After that, they put on another night sister, so the work was not quite so hard, and we could take rather longer spells in the duty room to get warm, but we have not had rain (as well as the cold) except on those two nights.

Last night was full of excitement: during the day a poor young Australian lad had gone off his head and had been put in a guard tent, and he tried to get hold of the sentry's bayonet. Then there was much commotion because the C.O. found one of the signalmen was drunk, and brought him down to the guard tent. Then Sister —— found an orderly straying about, who was supposed to be special with a young R.A.M.C. lieutenant who is down with fever, and the orderly did not seem to know what he wanted; so Sister flew off to the tent, and found the lieutenant very much upset, and saying that the orderly was quite mad, and had refused to go and fetch the wardmaster when he ordered him to do so; he said he could not tell Sister what mad things the orderly had been doing; so she had to send for the medical officer, who got the orderly removed at once and another posted.

There is not nearly so much drinking as there was at first, but still they do find ways of getting drunk at times. A little while ago there was a great row because the convalescent officers were allowed to drive or ride about, and they used to go over to the next town and bring back whisky and champagne. I don't think there was much harm in it at first (except that it was a bad example for the men), and it was winked at for some time, until they had a very rowdy lot of men in, and then one day one of them was found to be suffering from D.T.

I am glad I am not Lady Superintendent up here: I should find it hard to know where to draw the line with the present lot of sisters; at first they were given every liberty, and were rather encouraged to go to dances and riding picnics, &c., with the men; then, when their behaviour began to be talked about, the authorities put up notices in our mess-room of rules referring to conduct of which no lady would be guilty, rules which were, in fact, an insult to us, but which we cannot say are unnecessary, because there are just a few sisters who don't care what they do—one of them was seen at a hotel at the next station smoking cigarettes with a most undesirable companion!

We can only hope the war will soon be over, and let us all go home; otherwise, the sooner sisters of that sort are weeded out the better. They seem to have been choosing the sisters in a very casual way at home lately, and, though there are plenty of sisters out here who are working hard and well, they will probably all get classed together in the public estimation with those who are simply "frivolling" and getting themselves talked about.

XLVII

It is a long time since I have written to you, but for some time things went jogging on very much the same as when I wrote last, and there was little to write about, and then lately I have had a wretched time of it, so did not feel inclined for writing.

After I finished my turn on night duty I went back to my line, but soon knocked up, and was ill and off duty for nearly three weeks; first with dysentery, and then my damaged side got bad again.

By the time I got to work once more, the weather had very much improved, and my tents were very light. I received from home some splendid boxes of literature, and also of tobacco and jerseys, and some games for the men. I taught them to play Halma, and it was very popular; they used to make out it was a competition between the different branches of the Service—the greens were always the Volunteers, the yellows were the Yeomanry, the reds the Regulars, and the blues the Navy or the Colonials; sometimes they could get a representative of each branch to play the men, and then there was much excitement as to which would get in first.

The men in my line got a photographer to photograph them, and presented me with a large copy. You can understand that we were fairly slack when I tell you that we used to brew toffee in the duty room on afternoon duty. I think we were all very tired of ration feeding, and we were all getting thin, and when one gets to that stage one has a sort of craving for sweet things, so the toffee was very popular.

Something went wrong with the washing arrangements for a time, and we could not get our things washed, so for a week or two we had to wash for ourselves, and, irons being very scarce, we had to press our things by putting them under our mattresses and sleeping on them!

A column camped for a night near to us, and sent us in some sick, including a good many cases of measles, that had to be sent to an Isolation Camp. They had no sisters out there, and it was pretty rough and very dull; but the provision cart went out every day, so I was often able to send them parcels of papers, &c.

Early in September the Town Guard were all under arms, as there was some looting of stock quite near to us; and there were many rumours that we were going to be attacked (for the sake of the rifles and ammunition that the patients had brought in). The rifles, &c., were therefore sent to the next station.

After that there was more fighting down at Dundee, and then the Natal Volunteers were ordered out again.

All this time I was very seedy, and trying to exchange to another station; but several of us had rather good reason to believe that, so many sisters having sent in for an exchange, their applications were never forwarded to the P.M.O.!

Then they had a "Court of Inquiry" at the hospital, and I was obliged to give some evidence: and it was simply horrid having to do so. After that I felt so bad I wrote to the P.M.O. direct to say that as I could not get an exchange, might I be allowed to resign? as my brother was just now in Natal, and I proposed to go to stay with him, before going to England.

At last I obtained leave of absence, and later on obtained leave to resign.

Very much to my surprise, about this time, I learnt that I had been "mentioned in despatches," and, a little later on, that I had been awarded the Royal Red Cross; I am sure I have not done anything to earn it, nor have I done as much as many of the others; but, of course, it is very nice all the same.

I had such an awfully kind letter of farewell from the men of my line before I left, thanking me for what I had done for them.

We had a good many "Gentlemen Troopers" in, the last part of my time, and some exceedingly nice fellows amongst them. One, who was especially helpful, had been an officer on one of the big liners that came out here, before the war. He is now a gunner on one of the armoured trains, and has had a very exciting time of it.

My brother was in Durban, so I left one morning at 3 A.M. to join him; I put myself to bed in the train the night before, but I was prevented from sleeping by the shunting of engines and by the letting off of steam, &c. I was the only lady on the train till we had got some way down the line. We were delayed for an hour soon after we had started, as there had been a bad collision the day before, and as the telegraph line was damaged they had to give us a pilot engine.

It was a very rough line, and the train swayed about so tremendously that I was feeling quite sea-sick; then, when we were rattling down a steep hill, there was a sudden explosion, which, of course, made us think of Boers and many things, and we pulled up with such terrific jerks that we and our baggage all became mixed up on the floor. As soon as we could disentangle ourselves, we looked out—quite expecting to see a party of Boers—but only saw one man waving his arms violently, and we came to a standstill just as we rounded a sharp curve, and found ourselves immediately on the tail of a heavy coal train that had got stuck on our line; the explosion was a fog signal they had laid to stop us, and it saved us from coming a very nasty cropper down a steep bank.

I had told my brother I should spend the night with friends at Pinetown and join him in Durban the next day; but when I was leaving I had a wire from him to say I had better come straight down, as he might have to sail the next day, so, *en route*, I wired to my friends not to expect me.

I had a very early breakfast at Glencoe (and the usual wash at a tap on the platform!), and we were so late in reaching Estcourt, where we were supposed to lunch, that by that time I had a really bad headache, and could only rise to a cup of tea and a roll.

Inchanga is the place where one always dines, whether going up or down, and we were due there about 7 P.M., but about 8.30 P.M. we got stuck in a siding about a mile from Inchanga; and there we had to remain nearly an hour because Lord Milner was dining at Inchanga, and we had to wait till he had passed; we did not bless him for taking so long over his dinner while we starved! By this time I was feeling really ill, and thought it might be partly from want of food, so I made myself eat some soup and a little chicken; then I was establishing myself in the train again (thankful to think that it was a "no stop" run to Durban), when another wire was thrust into my hand from my brother saying, "No beds, if possible sleep Pinetown; not leaving till following day." I groaned, but bundled out again, with my kit-bag open, and my rugs, pillow, books, &c., all loose, just as the train departed. I thrust my goods into the hands of an astonished little Kaffir boy, who helped me to pack up my kit-bag, and of course I had to leave my heavy baggage to take care of itself.

I did not have to wait long for the "Kaffir Mail," which *does* stop at Pinetown, but I knew my friends would all have gone to bed as they were not expecting me, and of course no one would meet the train, and their house was some way from the station, and it was raining steadily! so I felt pretty miserable. I was put in a carriage by myself, and after we had started found there was no light in it, and I felt really ill, and wished I had not made myself eat any dinner!

However, just as we ran into Pinetown I looked out, and some one hailed me, and there was one of my best old Pinetown orderlies (now working on the line). He seemed so pleased to see me that I felt inclined to embrace him, but refrained! As soon as he had seen the train off and had locked up the station, he shouldered my bag and escorted me to my friend's house. They were all fast asleep, but soon let me in, and I don't know when I have been so thankful to turn into a comfortable bed as I was that night. It was a little over eight months since I had slept in a house.

The next morning they brought me a delicious breakfast in bed—hot scones, &c.; you don't know what it was like after camp feeding, to have a pretty tray with a cloth on it, and everything dainty and nice; and I was very loth to leave both my bed and my kind friends; but about mid-day I again boarded the train for Durban, retrieved my baggage at the station, and then found my brother at the Marine Hotel.

I had time to see a few friends and do a little very necessary shopping, and then we went on board the *Arundel Castle* to go down the coast to Port Elizabeth.

You can't think how funny it was to walk upstairs again: the Pinetown house was a bungalow, so I did not have to try stairs till I got on board ship. I still feel as though I must duck my head every time I go through a door, and when it blows in the night I always wake up and wonder whether I ought to take the mallet and attend to the tent-pegs; and then, when I realise I am not under canvas, there is such a satisfaction in being able to lie down and go to sleep again.

We did not stay in Port Elizabeth, but travelled by train straight on here, where my brother has about three days' work. We have a very comfortable little house to ourselves, with a garden full of such lovely flowers— Maréchal Niel roses, &c.

This is a pretty little town, and many of the people, who are most pleasant and friendly, have called on me. Near to Uitenhage there are still some wild elephants, but I had not time to make their acquaintance.

To-day the minister of the Dutch Reformed Church took us to see the Riebeck Girls' College; such good buildings, and such bright-looking scholars. They have a kindergarten, and then all the standards up to the highest—those working for university exams. The Resident Magistrate took us to see some nursery gardens that send flowers all over South Africa. After the barrenness of the Natal uplands these masses of flowers were quite lovely, and I was given a beautiful bunch of carnations.

To-night we have some people dining with us, and to-morrow we return to Port Elizabeth, where we shall probably stay about ten days.

XLVIII

From Uitenhage we returned to Port Elizabeth, where my brother had about a week's work, and then we had to wait a few more days for a steamer; but several old Kimberley friends were down there, and a good many other people called, so I had a very pleasant time.

Port Elizabeth was a little agitated about the plague; they had had about a hundred cases, and about half of that number had died, but just then there were only twelve in the hospital.

One day I went out with three ladies to a place they call the Red House, and had a delightful row up the Zwartkops River. Another day Mrs. —— drove my brother and me out to her father's country house, "Kraggakama," about a fourteen mile drive; a beautiful bungalow house, and such a lovely garden, surrounded by dense, semi-tropical woods, with little paths leading away into the woods; many monkeys and other creatures around.

We had lunch out there, and found strawberries just ripe in the garden.

From Port Elizabeth we had meant to go straight back to Kimberley, but, after many wires, it was decided that my brother must go to Oudtshoorn, a place a long way from the railway, where there had been cases waiting for a long time for trial, as it had not been considered safe for a judge to travel there.

To reach Oudtshoorn it was necessary to go by steamer to Mossel Bay, and the mail steamers, as a rule, do not call at Mossel Bay. Moreover, Port Elizabeth being an infected port (with plague), the mail steamers were not keen on taking passengers from there; so there were many obstacles to be overcome.

I packed up my heavy baggage and sent it up to Kimberley; then the *Norman* was signalled, and we went down to the jetty, and had to be examined by the medical officer of health for plague symptoms! and then the harbour-master took us off in a special tug.

The next morning they put us ashore at Mossel Bay, and there we had to wait some hours as the Commandant was very doubtful as to which was the safest route for us to take; there were still a good many Boers in the surrounding country, and, though they probably would not wish to interfere with us, they would certainly be very pleased to annex our provision cart and also our horses and mules; and the C.O. had so weak a garrison that he could spare us only a small escort.

After some time spent in wiring, it was decided we should drive to George and sleep there. The baggage and provisions were sent on with a mule cart, and, after an early lunch, we got away in two Cape carts with four horses each.

The distance was about thirty miles, and we outspanned only once—at Brak River, where we had some tea, and there an escort of six cyclists met us from George, and the Mossel Bay men turned back. The cyclists were very smart fellows; some of them scouted ahead, and the others rode with us very steadily uphill and down. It was getting dark when we neared George, and the Commandant and Magistrate rode out to meet us, and then stayed and had dinner with us at the hotel.

George is a pretty place, with streets lined with fine old oaks, and with big arum lilies growing in the fields around.

Just in front of the hotel there was a stout little sandbag fort with a small gun, and, of course, there was very strict "Martial Law" there; pickets on every road, and no one could leave the village or come in without a permit, and even with a permit you must be within the picket lines by sundown. No one might be outside his house after 9 P.M., and lights must be all out by 10 P.M.

We were to sleep at George, and the Commandant told us that he had already sent out a patrol of men, who were to sleep at the top of the Montague Pass, and meet us there the next morning; he wished us to slip away quietly in the early morning, and his patrol would soon join us, and ride with us till we met the troop that was being sent out from Oudtshoorn to meet us.

The Commandant has about 300 men under him. They are nearly all local men, in fact many of them Boers, but he was quite confident of their loyalty, and said the poor chaps were suffering badly for it, the rebels burning their farms and doing them all the harm they possibly could. Just when we were there he was very sad because one of his scouts, quite a young lad belonging to George (and very popular in the place), had been most cruelly shot by them after he had had to surrender.

The next day we started in our carts about 6.30 A.M., every one seeming to think it would be a risky drive. After we had gone some way our driver began to pull up and looked scared (he could speak only Dutch), and we made out that he could see some horses off-saddled higher up the mountain, and he thought it was Boers waiting for us. With some difficulty we explained to him that we expected the George escort to meet us at the beginning of the Pass, and then he agreed to go on; but we were all somewhat relieved when we got up to the horses and found they belonged to genuine District Mounted Troops, and that they had not seen any Boers about.

That day we travelled between forty and fifty miles, through beautiful mountain scenery, which reminded us of Switzerland (minus the snow); lovely ferns and cool, dripping water, and quite high mountains all round.

We outspanned only once for a breakfast-lunch at Doom River about 10 A.M.; Scheeper's commando had honoured them with a visit there, for looting purposes, just before he was caught.

At Hymen's House, about mid-day, we were met by a captain and twenty-two men from Oudtshoorn, and the George men went back. We got safely into Oudtshoorn about 3 P.M., and expected to be there about three or four days, but the work was heavier than had been expected, and we were there a whole fortnight. This was rather fortunate for me, as I knocked up with a very sharp touch of dysentery again, and should not have been fit to travel much sooner.

The Oudtshoorn people were extremely kind, and, when I got better, I had some charming drives to visit farms and other places of interest. It is a rich farming district, and it was the first time I had seen anything of ostrich farming and tobacco growing; so I found a great deal to interest me; they also grow grapes and other fruits, and it is a good corn-growing country.

The ostriches do especially well all along the course of the Oliphant's River. I got some good photos of the ungainly creatures.

Martial law was very strict, and (besides the same rules as those which I told you were in force at George) the farmers were not allowed to keep any horses or food supplies on their farms in case the Boers should take a fancy to them;—all horses had to be sold to the Remount Department at a fixed price, and farmers and other residents in the district, who were accustomed to keeping plenty of good horses, might be seen coming into town with oxen in their traps; and as they were not allowed to keep more than a week's supply of food or forage on their farms, and as some lived many miles away, they had to spend a good part of their time on the road in drawing their rations, as, of course, the oxen are very slow travellers.

They were reaping the corn when we were there, and it all had to be carted into town and sold to the military people, as they cut it.

Oudtshoorn, being far from the railway, had been very short of provisions (groceries, &c.) for some time past, and the military authorities would not allow any waggons to go up from the coast without a strong escort (which could not often be spared); but a convoy had been sent through before we got there, so there was plenty of food, and our provision cart had a few luxuries which seemed to be appreciated at the two dinner parties we gave.

From Oudtshoorn we still had more than a day's journey to join the railway at Prince Albert Road, and horses were so scarce that it was not easy to get decent animals. We sent the baggage cart (with mules) on ahead, and, eventually, my brother and I (and our man) got away in a light Cape cart with two fairly good horses, and the other men had four screws in a bigger cart. The scenery, as we crossed the Zwartberg, was very *grand*, but not quite so *pretty* as the Montague Pass. It was very stiff work for the horses, and we walked a good deal. Our first outspan was near the Cango Caves, where they had recently had a visit from a Boer commando; and then we had to give the horses a good rest at the "Victoria Hotel," high up on the Zwartberg.

We were rather disturbed to find, when we caught up our baggage cart, that it had no brake on it: the road is tremendously steep, as it zigzags down the mountain; so the sergeant in charge of our escort left a trooper to help the boy bring the mules down.

We got in about 7 P.M., but there was no sign of the baggage cart that night, and the Commandant (who had ridden out to meet us and then dined with us) was anxious, because only one trooper had been left with it, so he sent some more men out to meet them.

We had to go to bed without our baggage, feeling very anxious, as every one seemed to think the Boers would much like to get hold of it, and also of the mules.

I have seen plenty of barbed wire in South Africa, but have never seen so much as at Prince Albert; they stretch it even across the village street at night, and you can't go many yards without getting tied up in it.

The next morning, if we were to catch our train (and there was only the one train a day), we knew we must be away by 7.30 A.M.; but still no sign of our baggage; and then, at last, we heard that it was safe, but the crossbar of the harness had broken, and they had had to spend the night on the top of the mountain; a trooper had ridden in and gone back with new harness; so, after sitting at our gate with the Commandant, with a fresh supply of carts, and a fresh escort, until it was too late for it to be *possible* for us to catch our train, we had to decide to wait till the next day, and various wires had to be despatched about the railway carriage, &c.

About two hours later the missing baggage-cart arrived all well, with a very weary driver and troopers in attendance.

We had a pleasant day at Prince Albert, and the next day (having sent the baggage on at an early hour) we had an easy drive of twenty-eight miles with some excellent horses (most kindly lent to us by the Commandant), to the rail at Prince Albert Road. We outspanned only once, at Boter's Kraal, where the final escort met us, the sergeant coming up to salute and to tell us that he and his men "had searched the kopjes thoroughly since 4 A.M., and had seen no Boers to-day!" but at Boter's Kraal they told us of a recent visit from Pyper's commando.

Thus ended our 150 (odd) miles of driving across the Colony in this "sort of a war," without once having had the excitement of seeing any armed or hostile Boers. About thirty hours in a hot and dusty train brought us into Kimberley.

The dull old Karroo country looked much the same as when I saw it ten years ago, except that every few hundred yards on the line a blockhouse is standing, and a sentry in his shirtsleeves marches up and down with his rifle, while the rest of the garrison (some half-dozen men) come to look at the train, and to sing out "Papers." They have a terribly monotonous life, and one throws them every scrap of literature one possesses.

XLIX

I think it is just about ten years since I was here last; and *how* the place has changed! Many of my old friends have left, and so many have died that I am beginning to be almost afraid to ask after any one in case I should hear of his death.

Of course they have been through all the horrors of a four months' siege, and there are still many marks of the Boer shells to be seen; one of them had made a hole through our backyard wall and buried itself in the kitchen wall: Peter (the cat) found this hole very convenient when going out to visit his friends.

Many people still preserved the bombproof shelters or "dug-outs" in their gardens, where they used to take refuge when the shelling was going on, and then go back into their houses at night to cook the food, &c.

There is a big steam hooter at De Beers Mine, and, during the siege, whenever the lookout men saw the Boers preparing to shell the town, the hooter was sounded, and every one scuttled into shelter; and even now, whenever the hooter sounds, people start up and look inclined to run.

The civilians here cannot say enough for the way Mr. Cecil Rhodes worked during the siege; and his thoughtfulness and consideration for the women and children were beyond all praise. At one time he had many hundreds of them in safety down one of the mines, 1000 feet below the surface, and he took infinite pains to send them down suitable supplies; they were in fairly airy chambers, and had a good supply of electric light, &c. Of course the military people are not so enthusiastic about his assistance, but, naturally, they would not appreciate a man who always liked to have his own way, and do what he thought best—and who did it too!

The first thing the Boers did was to seize the waterworks, some miles from the town, and cut off the water supply; but the mine-owners came to the rescue by pumping water from a good spring in one of their mines that had caused them years of annoyance by rising and making the working of that mine a great difficulty; so the water question never caused them much trouble, though the Boers were constantly trying to damage the pumping machinery.

Though the water supply was fair the food supplies were very low; and a rich family, whom I know, told me they were intensely grateful to a neighbour who sent them a quarter of a bottle of port wine and half a packet of cornflour as a Christmas present. They were at that time drawing half their ration of meat in horseflesh, and, though some people say they could never touch it, I believe it was not at all bad, and one girl told me that a little donkey was "quite nice."

A good story is told of a colonel who was then up here. One night at mess he said, "Gentlemen, I am sorry to say we were only able to draw half our ration in beef to-day; this joint I am carving is beef, at the other end of the table the joint is horse: if any one would prefer to try it, perhaps he will carve for himself." No one got up, so the Colonel had to carve (small helpings) for all the mess. After they had finished an orderly came and whispered to him, and he said, "Oh, gentlemen, I am sorry to find I have made a mistake; I find this was the horse, and the cow is still at the other end of the table!"

There was so much sickness in the town that the doctors had a terrible time. In most cases it was suitable food rather than medicine that was needed, especially amongst the little children; and, besides the sickness, there were a great many wounded constantly being brought in from the trenches, or from skirmishes, and every available building was turned into a hospital.

I have just been reading Dr. Ashe's book, *Besieged by the Boers*, and it gives a good idea of the daily life up here, showing how men tried to go on and do their daily round of work in spite of the shells that were falling and killing not only men but women and children around them.

The thing that Kimberley people are most proud of is the big gun "Long Cecil," which was most cleverly designed and made in the De Beers workshops during the siege, the shells for it also being cast there; until that was built they had *no* guns of sufficient size to reply to the 100-pounder that the Boers were using with so much effect upon the town. It must have been a huge surprise to them when Long Cecil began to scatter shells amongst them, each one inscribed, "With C. J. R.'s compliments!"

The cemetery is sadly full of "siege" graves, and so many little children's graves amongst them. Strangely enough one of the De Beers engineers (an American) who was chiefly responsible for the building of "Long Cecil," was killed by a Boer shell only a few days after the gun was completed; and, just as an example of how we were surrounded by enemies even inside the town, I will tell you about his funeral.

In such a hot climate as South Africa it is always necessary that the funeral should take place within about twenty-four hours of the death; so that it is quite possible to be talking to a man in his shop or at his business in the morning, for him to be taken suddenly ill and die that evening, and the next day, before you have heard of his illness, for you to meet his coffin on the way to the cemetery.

Well, this poor engineer was a very popular man, and the Commandant thought that many people would wish to attend his funeral, so he gave directions that it should be at night, for safety from the Boer shells. Late in the evening, when it was quite dark, the funeral left the hospital; but it had no sooner started than a rocket was seen to go up *in* the town, evidently a pre-arranged signal—for almost at once the Boers began to drop shells around the cemetery, but fortunately no one was killed.

Perhaps you have heard in England of the little girl who knew so much about martial law that she strayed into the Provost's office one day in December and said, "Please, sir, may I have a permit for Santa Claus to come to our house!"

All food seems to be frightfully expensive still: we have to pay about 8s. for a single fowl or duck, 4s. a dozen for eggs, and 2s. 6d. a pound for butter.

We have a white woman as cook, and our black boy rejoices in the name of "Moses." I had not been here many days before "George" came to see me— the boy I used to have ten years ago. It is extraordinary how these natives know when one returns, even years afterwards. Of course George wanted to come back, but I found he was in a good place, so I told him I was soon going back to England, and I did not take him on.

I have had two offers of rather good posts out here, but I think I must go home for a time at any-rate.

There is a huge refugee camp just outside Kimberley. I am afraid they have had an awful lot of measles in these camps, and there have been many deaths from it; measles were almost unknown on the scattered Boer farms, and now that these people are crowded together in close quarters, with their traditional objection to fresh air or cleanliness, it seems impossible to make them take precautions against infection.

As a rule, the people in the refugee camps have rations quite as good, and often much better, than the troops, but they do not thrive on them; still, it was impossible to leave them on the farms, for the only way to prevent the Boers from keeping up their supplies was to take or destroy the crops, and, after that was done, it was impossible to leave the women and children on the farms to starve.

Now they are sending sisters to work in these camps, and they are doing all they can to help the people, but I fancy it must be rather uphill work, as many of the Boer women are so very suspicious and bitter. I daresay you have heard of the woman who urged her husband to go and fight, saying, "I can get another husband, but I can't get another Free State."

I have had some interesting drives round the country with a lady who was here all through the siege, and could show me where the fighting had taken place; and one day some officers gave a very jolly picnic at a place called "The Bend," about seventeen miles from here, on the Vaal River.

It was very hot weather just then, 90° to 95° in the shade, so we started at 5.30 A.M., and had breakfast and lunch out there. A mulecart loaded with provisions—delicious peaches and other fruits which had been sent up from Cape Town—had been despatched in charge of four orderlies (all armed). We rowed on the river and prowled about under the trees; and altogether it was quite the nicest picnic I have ever enjoyed.

One of the officers of our party had the honour of being the youngest Colonel in the British Army; he has been promoted so rapidly during the war.

They had all had a rough time of hardship, but they meant to enjoy themselves that day, and I think they did; but they kept their revolvers handy even when rowing up the river.

I had been told that I was entitled to an "Indulgence Passage" home, as I have served during the war, and that would mean that I should have to pay only about £5 for my mess on a trooper, instead of paying about £35 for a passage on an ordinary mail-boat; so I went to the railway staff officer, and he was most kind in arranging about it for me, and (after communicating with Cape Town) he told me that if I would see the P.M.O. when I arrived down there, he would probably be glad if I would do duty for the voyage, and then I could travel quite free, and receive pay (instead of having to pay my mess bill). He also gave me a free railway pass down to the Cape, which I had not at all expected.

Now, I must pay some farewell calls; and then, once more, I shall soon be on the move again.

It really does seem as though the war will soon be over now. We hear that some troops are still coming out, but there appear to be more than enough sisters for the work that has to be done.

L

S.S. "ORIENT" (*en route* for HOME),
March 1902.

I was very sorry to say good-bye to Kimberley, but I was also getting very home-sick, so early one morning I once more joined the train, to stroll across the Karroo and down to Cape Town.

I had armed myself with a large stock of literature, kindly given to me by friends, and also by the librarian of the Kimberley Public Library (who gave me a noble stock of back numbers), and this I distributed to the men at the blockhouses on the way. Poor fellows, they have a trying time of it, they must be very wide awake and alert, or any night the Boers may cross the section of line for which they are responsible, very likely leaving a little dynamite to wreck the next train; and yet for weeks and perhaps months never a Boer may come near their particular section.

The trains were still not supposed to travel at night, so we tied up about 6 P.M. on the first day at De Aar. After dinner I was just thinking it was very slow, not knowing any one in the place, and I thought I would go to bed, when I saw a General strolling along the platform, and with him a young officer whom I soon recognised as an old Pinetown patient, and whom I was very glad to meet again.

The General soon departed, and then Captain —— took me for a jolly moonlight walk round De Aar; he was still a little lame from his wound, so was acting as Adjutant for some Yeomanry there. It was pleasant to hear about many other old friends, and also a little about the course of the war in that part of the country.

The next day, as we proceeded down the line, we passed some troop trains going up with men who had just arrived fresh from England—I think some of the Scots Guards, the Manchesters, and the Lancashire Fusiliers. Some of them were tightly packed in open waggons, and appeared to think they were having a rough time already, but, as the weather was warm and dry, they were not so badly off. They seemed very glad of the few papers which I could give them, as they had seen none since they landed. Their chief anxiety seemed to be as to whether they would have the chance of firing off a little ammunition before the war is over.

That night we tied up at Matjesfontein, and I much regretted I could not stay a day there to explore the battlefield; but I did not know which day they wanted me for duty, so I had to hasten on.

The next morning I arrived in Cape Town; and, after a "wash and brush up," I went to see the P.M.O., who was most kind, and said that if I was willing to do light duty on the voyage, I certainly need not pay for a passage. If I was ready, he would like me to go on board the *Orient* on the 12th (it was then the 8th).

I had a few very pleasant days with some friends at Rondebosch; but I was unable to get about much to see other people, as I was again very seedy with dysentery, and had to doctor myself rather severely in order to get ready for duty on the 12th.

I came on board that morning at 10 A.M., but there was such a gale blowing that we did not get away till 5 P.M. the next day.

There are about thirty officers and between 500 and 600 men on board, almost all of them invalided home, and it is awfully sad to see so many "wrecks" of the war.

The P.M.O. is a major of the R.A.M.C., and he is just as strict with the orderlies as the major I worked with at Pinetown; so the men are well cared for, and I am enjoying working for him.

I was the first sister to join the ship, and, as I found the cabins would be very full, I asked if I might act as night sister, and thereby I secured a cabin to myself.

I have had plenty to do most of the way, as there have been several men and one officer very ill all the time; but we have had no deaths on the voyage, and most of the patients seem to be mending now.

On my first night on duty I had been round the hospital, and then I thought I would take a look at the convalescent men in the swinging cots (ninety of them), and I found there a poor colour-sergeant, who had been out only a few months, going back with hopelessly bad heart disease from overstrain; he was unable to lie down, and so breathless and blue, I got him transferred to the hospital, and was able to make him comfortable with pillows, &c. He has been such a good patient and has improved a little, but I fear he can never work again, and he is a married man.

There are two quite young lads who have been having epileptic fits frequently on the voyage—I suppose brought on by exposure to the South African sun.

A young Yorkshire farmer of the Yeomanry was invalided home as a "phthisis" case, but he came into hospital the day after we sailed with a temperature of 105°, and he has been desperately ill with enteric all the way (severe hæmorrhage, &c.). He must have had fever for some time before it was diagnosed—the temperature being attributed to his chest condition. He is still very weak, but I think he will pull through.

One night I was told that a man in the swinging cots was "rather peculiar," so I went down to see him first thing, and found his cot empty. I flew up on deck, and met some stewards, who had collared him on the upper deck. We made him snug in a safe corner of the hospital with a "special" for that night. Then, there was one poor fellow who had lost an arm, and two who had each lost a leg—one of the latter a sergeant-major, who was wounded at the same time that Colonel Benson was killed at Vlakfontein. He was a Kimberley man, and the poor man's wife and two little children were all killed by one Boer shell during the siege of Kimberley. He is going home to get fitted up with a cork leg, and will then return to South Africa.

Perhaps the saddest cases of all were the eleven lunatics we had on board. They had to be very safely kept with special guards and other precautions; and, in case they should try to go overboard, they had a high-railed enclosure on deck as an airing ground. Some of them are very mad and violent, but some seemed so nearly sane that it was a question whether they had not pretended to be mad in order to be sent home.

I was not supposed to visit these men in the night, because, to get to them, I should have had to go a long way through the troops' sleeping quarters, but the medical officer went to see them on his last round, and, every two or three hours, I used to stay in the hospital while the wardmaster went along, and brought word how they were.

One night the medical officer went along, and when he returned he told me he had found their door unlocked and no guard on duty; fortunately they were all asleep. The next day this tale was about the ship, and very soon it was altered to the following version—"Last night Mr. —— had found that all the lunatics had escaped; he and Sister thought it better not to make a fuss. Instead, they caught the first eleven men whom they met and locked them up; they were not the *real* lunatics, but they had been bribed with extra 'skoff' to play the game and say nothing about it: but the real lunatics were still at large!" After that, if any one came up to a man rather quietly, there was a big jump, and "Hullo! are you one of them?" and then a great chase round the deck!

There were some hard cases, too, amongst the officers; two of them who had thighs broken by Boer shells, but were just beginning to walk again—one, however, with a short leg, and the other with a stiff knee.

A Yeomanry officer, badly shot in both arms, had one hand still quite useless; but I hope an operation may improve matters. He had had a dreadful time in the jolting ambulance waggons, unable to hold on, or to save himself with either hand.

Then, there was a young doctor who once, when our men were surprised and many of them taken, was going round dressing the wounded, when some Boers came up and shot the wounded as he was dressing them, and afterwards led him out several times saying they were going to shoot him, but eventually he got safely away. There were two officers shot through the lungs, but I think they will recover in time; and there was another young fellow shot in the region of the spine, and paralysed all down one side and leg; and yet another (quite a boy) shot in the thigh and paralysed on that side. Neither of these two could move without assistance; and, though they were all wonderfully bright and cheerful, I know I often found them lying awake for hours together, and it is hard for a young Englishman to face the thought that he may never be able to walk or ride again, even when he *has* received his wound in defence of his country.

As I finish this letter, we are just anchoring for the night in Southampton Water, off Netley Hospital; and, curiously enough, it is March 3rd, the very day I sailed for South Africa two years ago. To-morrow we hope to land at Southampton.

After a little time at home, I hope to persuade a sister of mine to pay a visit with me to another brother in the United States, and to some relations in Canada and Nova Scotia; then I must settle down to some steady work in England.

I would not have missed nursing through this war for a great deal. We have often had rough times, and anxious times, and of course I have not been able to do much, but I have been able to help a few men to recover their health and strength; and, perhaps, also to help a few in their last hours, men whose own relations would have given much to have been in my place, where it was not possible for them to be. And, however busy I was, I could at least find time to remind them that ... "God shall wipe away all tears from their eyes; and there shall be no more death, neither sorrow, nor crying, neither shall there be any more *pain*." ...

Still no one, who has not seen it, can realise the sorrow and the suffering that war entails; and I am *almost* inclined to agree with a man who was in Kimberley during the siege, who helped Mr. Cecil Rhodes in his work there, and who afterwards, when asked if he was not glad that he had had the chance of assisting Mr. Rhodes in his great work, said, "Yes, but when I think of all the suffering those unfortunate women and children had to endure, I think if I was ever again in a country where war was imminent, I should take a ship to the other side of the world, and stop there till it was over!"

I fear that we are not likely all to be able to do that; but I trust this war will have had the effect of making people think, and that should there ever be another war in our time, we may be better prepared for it.

War must always mean suffering, but the suffering might be enormously lessened if we were better organised in times of peace.